Recruitment and Retention of Substance-Using Pregnant and Parenting Women

Lessons Learned

Marilyn Poland Laken, Ph.D., R.N.
Ellen Hutchins, Sc.D., M.S.W.

Supported by
Maternal and Child Health Bureau
Health Resources and Services Administration
Public Health Service
U.S. Department of Health and Human Services

Published by
National Center for Education in Maternal and Child Health
Arlington, Virginia

Cite as
Laken MP, Hutchins E. 1996. *Recruitment and Retention of Substance-Using Pregnant and Parenting Women: Lessons Learned.* Arlington, VA: National Center for Education in Maternal and Child Health.

The mission of the National Center for Education in Maternal and Child Health is to promote and improve the health, education, and well-being of children and families by leading a national effort to collect, develop, and disseminate information and educational materials on maternal and child health; and by collaborating with public health agencies, voluntary and professional organizations, research and training programs, policy centers, and others to advance knowledge in programs, service delivery, and policy development. Established in 1982 at Georgetown University, NCEMCH is part of the Graduate Public Policy Program. NCEMCH is funded primarily by the U.S. Department of Health and Human Services through its Maternal and Child Health Bureau.

Library of Congress Catalog Card Number 96-69415
ISBN 1-57285-033-7

Published by:
National Center for Education in Maternal and Child Health
2000 15th Street North, Suite 701
Arlington, VA 22201-2617
(703) 524-7802
(703) 524-9335 fax
Internet: ncemch01@gumedlib.dml.georgetown.edu
World Wide Web: http://www.ncemch.georgetown.edu

Single copies of this publication are available at no cost from:
National Maternal and Child Health Clearinghouse
2070 Chain Bridge Road, Suite 450
Vienna, VA 22182-2536
(703) 821-8955
(703) 821-2098 fax

This publication has been produced by the National Center for Education in Maternal and Child Health under its cooperative agreement (MCU-117007) with the Maternal and Child Health Bureau, Health Resources and Services Administration, Public Health Service, U.S. Department of Health and Human Services.

Table of Contents

Acknowledgments

The authors gratefully acknowledge the 10 project representatives from the Pregnant and Postpartum Women and Their Infants (PPWI) demonstration grant initiative who participated in the two-day focus group that resulted in this document. The participants gave generously of their time and willingly shared information gained from developing programs and services for pregnant and parenting substance-using women. We thank each of them for participating in a most informative focus group. Special thanks to Valerie Gwinner from the National Center for Education in Maternal and Child Health for providing logistical support for the focus group and for her assistance in the preparation of this monograph. We also appreciate the help of Gayle Vandenberg who provided assistance during the focus group.

Chapter 1

Introduction

Although drug use in America has been a serious social problem for decades, drug use among pregnant women was not widely reported as a public health problem until the mid-1980s. According to current national estimates, approximately 5.5 percent of all pregnant women use an illicit drug during pregnancy.[1]

Heroin use among pregnant women has been reported for years. Over the last decade women of childbearing age have used alcohol, marijuana, and heroin in relatively stable patterns. Cocaine, which is highly addictive, has become popular with women of childbearing age in recent years. The explosive increase in this population's use of the crystallized form of cocaine called "crack" has been viewed as responsible for dramatic increases in the number of infants born exposed to drugs.[2]

Prior to the introduction of crack cocaine and its frequent use by some women, drug use was seen as a disorder affecting primarily men. For that reason, few drug treatment programs were designed specifically for women, especially for pregnant women and mothers of young children. However, national concern for drug-exposed infants prompted interest in the needs of substance-using pregnant women and, thus, in the development of drug treatment programs for them.

In 1989, Congress appropriated funds for a comprehensive demonstration grant program called the Pregnant and Postpartum Women and Their Infants (PPWI) program. The Center for Substance Abuse Prevention (CSAP) of the Substance Abuse and Mental Health Administration (SAMHSA), with assistance from the Maternal and Child Health

Bureau (MCHB) of the Health Resources and Services Administration (HRSA), funded 147 projects under this program. This initiative is the largest federal program targeting pregnant substance-using women and their infants.

Some of the important findings from this federal program have been studied in two ways: (1) Each project conducted a local evaluation, and (2) a cross-site evaluation examined data among selected projects. Although findings from local and cross-site evaluations have increased our knowledge about how to prevent and address substance use in this population, the need remains to highlight and summarize some of the lessons learned in selected areas of interest.

Therefore, in 1994, a focus group composed of project representatives from 12 PPWI projects that had ended or were close to ending was convened. The group examined lessons learned from the perspective of the client and the system, highlighting: (1) case management, (2) building systems of care, and (3) sustainability. The findings from this focus group were synthesized into a monograph, which has been disseminated within the field.[3]

Similarly, there is a need to summarize information learned in the areas of recruitment and retention of substance-using pregnant and parenting women. This monograph is the product of a second two-day focus group, held in October 1995, which brought together representatives from 10 PPWI projects to discuss strategies for recruitment and retention of pregnant and parenting substance-using women.

Prenatal care early in pregnancy, as well as care after delivery, increase a woman's likelihood of having a healthy infant. Therefore, recruitment and retention strategies are very important when targeting substance-using pregnant and parenting women. Additionally, pregnancy offers a unique opportunity to reach substance-using women, as they may be more motivated to seek treatment on behalf of their babies.[4]

Needs of Pregnant and Parenting Substance-Using Women

The topics of recruitment and retention were selected for in-depth examination because: (1) Pregnant and parenting substance-using women present unique challenges to providers who are attempting to identify and retain women in treatment; (2) there is little published literature on these topics; and (3) professionals in the field agree that recruitment and retention are ongoing problems.

Women who are pregnant and using substances have unique needs. These women are more likely to have been victims of sexual and physical abuse in childhood, to have a parent who abused drugs or alcohol, and to have been introduced to drugs by a male partner.[5,6] Although they may experience denial, psychosocial problems, and illegal lifestyles in common with many substance abusers, pregnant women who disclose their substance use bear the additional stigma of a behavior that the general public, including health professionals, views as harmful to the women, to their unborn children, and to their other children.[7,8]

Substance use by pregnant women is viewed as more serious than that by men or women who are not responsible for young children. As a result, substance-using pregnant women are more likely to be under scrutiny by local justice officials and departments of child protective services. These women may be under threat of losing their children and, in some states, of incarceration for delivering drugs to the unborn or newborn.[9] Many of these women are ashamed of their habits and their lifestyles; however, they may be reluctant to seek treatment because disclosure may jeopardize their families and their relationships with their male partners.

Further, making a commitment to treatment may be frightening to many because it brings new awareness and a change in life patterns and relationships. Careful assessments must precede activities related to counseling and treatment. For example, one focus group participant reported:

> *Many of the women in our program were with men who abused drugs. We had a caseworker who worked with our clients on issues related to their relationships with their male partners. This caseworker believed that the men represented a negative influence on the women's drug problems and she urged the women to leave their partners. Several women left our program after receiving this advice.*
>
> *Treatment for substance abuse is not like treatment for a broken leg. Substance abuse involves a family and other close relationships. You have to treat those relationships to treat the woman.*
>
> Margery Brooks

There is mixed evidence in the literature regarding barriers to drug treatment or refusal to treat when pregnancy is disclosed.[10,11] For example, a 1989 study of 78 drug treatment programs in New York City found that only 13 percent accepted low-income pregnant women who used crack.[12] A more recent study of 294 drug treatment programs in five cities found that by 1993 most programs, including those in New York, accepted pregnant women.[13] Dually diagnosed pregnant women present unique needs and many find appropriate treatment especially difficult to obtain.[14]

Recruitment and retention of substance-using pregnant and parenting women takes place within this sociocultural milieu. This monograph explores many of the challenges and obstacles successful programs face in recruiting and retaining women.

Focus Group Structure

In this two-day focus group, representatives from 10 PPWI demonstration projects shared their observations, experiences, and project findings to capture lessons learned about how best to recruit and retain substance-using pregnant and parenting women and their infants. The participants were regionally and ethnically diverse, and represented 10 programs that differed in approaches used and populations served. (See Appendix.)

Led by Drs. Laken and Hutchins, the group explored barriers to recruitment and retention, as well as successful and unsuccessful strategies. Areas of group disagreement were analyzed further to elucidate differences in program structure and function, client characteristics, or the perspective of the group member. Proceedings were taped and transcribed. Discussion content was categorized by topic area and summarized.

In this volume stories and quotes by group participants illustrate or further explain content areas. Comparisons with published literature are included where appropriate, although information on recruitment is scarce. Quantitative data from the 10 projects have been collected to describe the client population and to quantify, when possible, the numbers of clients recruited and length of enrollment. Evaluation of the factors that may explain differences in recruitment and retention has been included.

The following summary is not meant to be comprehensive or to represent the experiences of all 147 projects. Rather, it attempts to capture the diverse opinions of 10 experts in the field who, over the two-day discussion, were able to reach consensus on most issues. ■

Chapter 2

Recruitment

What Is Recruitment?

Recruitment was defined by the group as a dynamic process for engaging clients. It involves defining the target population; designing program approaches and activities to meet a continuum of needs; and organizing the system of referrals and outreach to agencies, partners, families, and the community.

Recruitment begins with identifying a population, identifying its needs, and meeting those needs by establishing a collaborative process with relevant agencies and institutions. Due to the complex nature of substance use by pregnant and parenting women, the number of community agencies collaborating will be large. Because each agency has a different perspective about the target population, programs are most effective when community agency representatives come together to design the program. Programs are more likely to be successful when systems building occurs early rather than later.[3] Community agencies also provide important information about the needs of pregnant and parenting women that guides program activities. Agency participation may change over time as the women's needs change or are made clearer.

Recruitment of substance users in research projects concludes that projects must be familiar with the lifestyle of the client population and understand their complex needs.[15] Chemically dependent families have unique characteristics that may profoundly affect the recruitment process. These characteristics include: (1) intermittent altered mental status secondary to the acute effects of alcohol and/or other drugs, (2) the often untreated health care problems inherent in the population (e.g., sexually transmitted diseases, AIDS), and (3) violence associated with the drug lifestyle.[15–18] Further, the illicit nature of substance-abusing families and their frequent changes of address necessitate a personal, one-on-one approach.[16]

Programs must be available—this may mean evenings and weekends—and accessible to the target population and to the agencies and individuals who are likely to refer clients. Programs for substance-using pregnant and parenting women must not exist in isolation, but must consider the community, family, and male partner in developing services.

Recruitment may mean that, in some cases, substance-using women are recruited before they are willing to engage in treatment programs. For example, a woman may be court mandated to a treatment program, but she may not necessarily be engaged in the treatment process. Most women drop in and out of treatment several times before they are ready for treatment. The focus group members discussed providing women with incentives to participate. There were no clear-cut rules or agreement on which approach was most effective. Focus group participants did agree that programs have to be flexible and patient in their approaches. When or why clients decide to engage in the process is unclear.

The first client that ever entered our program left immediately after intake. We thought we would never see her again. When she delivered, her male partner brought her clothes to her in the hospital, but he lost her left shoe. She came to us to for a matched pair of shoes, which we provided. The woman was so impressed that we would do that for her that she returned to our program and recruited other clients as well. Now who would have known that a shoe would be a recruitment strategy?

Stephen Ridley

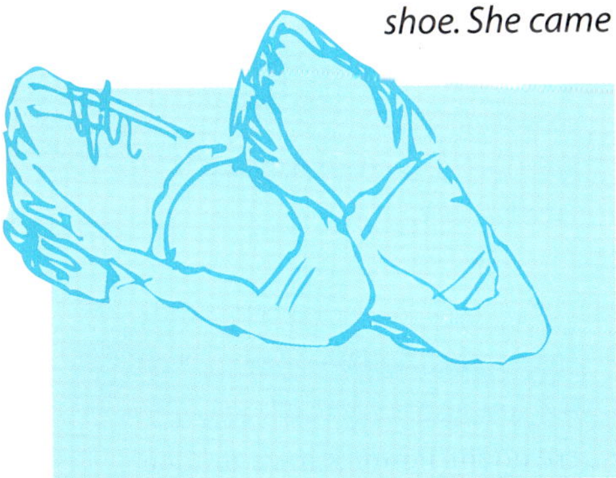

Recruitment Strategies

The 10 programs varied in the number of clients they recruited, from 106 to 401. Percentages of clients who were pregnant at the time of initial recruitment also varied from 21.7 percent to 98 percent. Differences in numbers recruited were due to the nature of the program, staff size, and success of the recruitment strategies used. Programs with intense case management and drug treatment followed fewer clients.

The group listed many recruitment strategies that they believed were effective. Some, such as establishing referral agreements, were easy to evaluate; others, such as making the program accessible to prospective clients, were more difficult to evaluate. Projects had varying successes with their recruitment strategies, and methods that may have worked in one site had limited success in another. The following approaches were used by many of the projects.

Referrals: One recruitment strategy that all of the projects used was getting referrals from outside agencies. Most focus group participants felt that this approach was their most successful, since substance-using women often sought care elsewhere in the system. Referrals were obtained through two approaches: building referral networks through community agencies, and promoting methods for screening patients for substance use in prenatal clinics and hospitals.

All projects began their programs by establishing a referral network among relevant agencies. Projects introduced themselves into the network of existing agencies by making presentations to agency staff and, in one case, preparing a resource directory.

> *Our project developed a resource directory with our logo on the front cover. The directory contained information about local agencies by category of need. For example, housing-related agencies were listed under that category. The directory was very popular and it helped everyone in the system. The resource directory is now being printed by another project. We assist with printing costs rather than duplicating this service.*
>
> JoAnne Lutz

Another project hired staff who had experience working in various established treatment programs. These staff members' knowledge of the agencies could link the new program with existing ones.

One project became involved with relevant agencies around a common problem—a local policy that automatically removed children from the mother if she was found to be using drugs. The project's advocacy on behalf of the women forged a bond with the existing system of providers. Several programs expressed the importance of monitoring the political climate within the community as it relates to substance-using pregnant women and within the system of providers. Becoming an active participant in the system and an advocate for substance-using pregnant women early in the life of the project fostered a clear identity and resulted in referrals.

Building systems of referrals often included addressing turf issues related to responsibility for the client. One project held monthly client review meetings where providers who referred women to the program could be kept informed about the progress of clients being case managed by the PPWI program. This approach addressed fears of community programs that the PPWI project would "take away" or somehow not address the needs of their clients. Hosting an open house for community agencies was another successful way to build relationships across agencies. Agencies often have one person who refers most of the clients. Inviting other staff from the same agency to the open house increased referrals from each agency.

Another strategy for reducing turf issues was to assist large agencies with their recruitment efforts. One program assisted in the effort to enroll pregnant women early in prenatal care, in hopes that screening for substance use in the prenatal clinic would result in referrals to the PPWI project. Program staff found that they first had to address negative attitudes of clinic staff toward substance-using pregnant women before the program received large numbers of referrals.

One project tried to form a network of collaborating agencies without success. Staff finally realized that they failed because they did not include the mayor's office—an office that was traditionally part of all coalitions in that area. The project felt it would have succeeded if it had done its homework and examined the existing network before proceeding on its own.

Several projects found that being available to help community agencies with their substance-using clients established trust in the new PPWI program and brought in many referrals. In community agencies, negative feelings about substance use were common. One program instituted small group and one-on-one discussions with agency staff to allow them to express their feelings about substance use. Often, community agency staff lived with family members who used substances and they needed to discuss their frustration and resulting negative attitudes toward clients who used. During one-on-one sessions, two staff members of community agencies admitted to using drugs, and the PPWI program referred them for treatment.

In two cases, projects that were linked with or housed in a hospital used that affiliation to establish referrals. For example, one program gained the cooperation of the nurses on the labor and delivery floor. The nurses called the program whenever a patient tested positive for drugs. Staff from the program would visit the patient to recruit her into the program. Program feedback to the nurses on the importance of this effort strengthened this referral link. Another PPWI program became part of a larger program in the same hospital. The larger program provided primary care for women at risk for HIV infection and poor pregnancy outcomes. The PPWI project took over the intake process and screened for drug use along with other risk factors. Thus, by becoming part of the larger program, they were able to obtain clients directly.

Other programs forged strong ties with large agencies outside of their institutions. One program had a letter of agreement with a local substance abuse clinic that gave referrals to the PPWI project in exchange for case management and transportation for eligible clients to return to the clinic. This relationship resulted in more than 400 referrals in the first three years of the project. Additionally, the transportation funded by the PPWI project helped retain clients in substance abuse treatment.

Another program obtained 24 percent of its referrals from the court system and another 10 percent from the local jail. Clients earned an early release from jail and went on probation if they agreed to enter the PPWI program. Some women preferred to go to jail "because it was less work." Several group members questioned the effectiveness of mandating treatment. Some women enter treatment only if they are mandated, and there was concern that these women would not become engaged in the treatment process.

Finally, several group members stressed the need for flexibility in referral networks. Most of the PPWI programs developed their recruitment strategies around finding women who used crack cocaine; this meant working with one set of referral agencies. When the drug of choice changed to heroin in some areas in the early 1990s, pregnant women began appearing in methadone treatment centers. This necessitated a switch in referral agencies. When a local methadone treatment agency was temporarily short of staff, one program helped dispense methadone in an effort to establish a stronger working relationship between the two agencies. The strategy worked, although the PPWI program had to reorient its staff to working with methadone maintenance.

Trying to reach physicians directly was one systems-building strategy that did not work. PPWI staff met with physicians to encourage them to attend small group conferences on screening methods or, in one case, a large interdisciplinary course on screening. One focus group member summed up the problem: "Doctors only listen to other doctors. They would not listen to us." This issue has arisen in other PPWI programs without resolution.[3] One group member suggested working with physicians at the departmental level to present screening methods through Grand Rounds and other hospital-based instruction. In this way, physicians would receive continuing medical education credits in their own learning environment.

Screening procedures: Another popular method of recruiting was to train clinic and hospital staff to screen pregnant and postpartum women for substance use. Seven of the 10 projects used this method. Three variations of promoting screening were described: (1) introducing a screening tool and conducting training on how to use it, (2) screening by the PPWI project staff, and (3) developing a tool in collaboration with a consortium of physicians for the purpose of statewide screening. The first variation was used by several programs. All group members agreed that screening was to be used for referral to appropriate services and not for imposing punitive sanctions. This was easiest to do when the PPWI project director also directed the state's maternity program.

> *Our statewide program initially used the Problem Oriented Pregnancy Risk Assessment System (POPRAS) prenatal record form for substance use screening in our maternity clinics. However, when we compared the number of women who admitted to substance use on the POPRAS with*

those who admitted they used with the Substance Abuse Subtle Screening Inventory (SASSI), we found four-fifths of the women who used when administering the POPRAS alone. Therefore, we trained our social work staff in the use of the SASSI. Social work staff would, in turn, train nursing staff how to screen clients. Pretests and posttests were used to document changes in knowledge of staff. Social workers would also observe clinic while clients were being screened and provided feedback to the nursing staff on how well they engaged clients. Staff felt this kind of feedback was very valuable to them in learning how to screen effectively.

Sally Carter

Some projects conducted training for certified nurse-midwives and physicians on how to screen for substance use. Several group members discussed initial reluctance on the part of hospital and clinic staff to become trained in assessment methods, suggesting that some nurses and physicians had negative attitudes toward substance-using pregnant women. This observation is supported by research on attitudes of health professionals.[19] However, one study reports that when certified nurse-midwives receive proper education and structural changes are made in care delivery, nurses' attitudes become more positive toward, and nurses become more effective in working with, substance-using pregnant women.[20]

During a focus group discussion led by the local evaluators in one program, clients said they felt physicians needed more training in how to screen for substance use. They also said that they would prefer to have physicians, rather than nurses or social workers, talk to them about their substance abuse problems. Some physicians agree. In a 1993 *Obstetrics and Gynecology* editorial, Richard Schwarz, M.D., pointed out that many obstetricians deny that their patients use substances and, consequently, do not screen their patients or prefer to have their office staff screen for substance use.[21] Additionally, while studies on the prevalence of substance use point to increased use in low-income populations, middle-income patients also use drugs in higher numbers than their physicians realize.[22]

One project developed a screening form for its program in collaboration with physicians. This form was integrated into a screening form that could be used in physician offices statewide. However, without support to train providers and support staff in its use, there was concern that the screening form would not be used or would be used incorrectly.

As mentioned above, another program actually performed substance abuse screening for a larger prenatal and high-risk program. This helped the prenatal program identify at-risk pregnant women and provided prospective clients for the PPWI project. One program had a social worker visit outside agencies and units within the hospital to remind staff about the PPWI program and to assist with screening. The project did not understand why this approach produced few referrals from outside agencies. One program adopted a reverse strategy—providing free pregnancy testing at substance abuse clinics. This helped identify pregnant women early in pregnancy and resulted in a limited number of referrals to the PPWI project.

Screening is an important way to identify substance use. A number of reliable screening instruments can be used to assess the woman's self-reported drug use. Self-reported drug use has been shown to be more accurate than urine toxicologies in some studies.[6,23] The most frequently used instruments for assessment of alcohol include the MAST (Michigan Alcoholism Screening Tool); the CAGE (Cut Down Annoyed Guilt Eye-opener) questionnaire; and the T-ACE (Tolerance Annoyed Cut Down Eye-opener).[24] One of the more common instruments for assessment of illicit drugs is a modified version of the Khavari instrument.[25]

Outreach: Outreach was defined by the group as an activity that goes beyond conventional program limits to connect the program to the needs of target populations. The target population was defined as clients, their families, related agencies, and the community.

Although seen as part of recruitment, outreach is primarily an educational process that may or may not directly bring clients into the program. For example, a video about substance use during pregnancy that contains the project name may be seen by an agency that then refers women to the project. Outreach efforts such as this are difficult to evaluate. Therefore, group participants were less sure of the effectiveness of most outreach strategies.

One commonly mentioned practice among 7 of the 10 programs was street outreach, which involves using program staff to visit places where prospective clients are likely to spend time. This may include Laundromats, clinics, local Special Supplemental Nutrition Program for Woman, Infants and Children (WIC) offices, beauty shops, bars, and stores. A few programs sent outreach workers door to door to post information in local stores as a way to reach prospective clients. One project used social workers ("dressed as public health nurses because it was safer") to visit women in their homes. After one social worker was inadvertently involved in a drug arrest, the program registered the cars of its outreach staff with the police. Some projects hired specially trained outreach workers, while others used case managers.

There are few published evaluations of the effectiveness of outreach workers in recruitment. While some report modest success, outreach efforts are seen as labor intensive and may not be cost-effective.[26] One project evaluated the extent to which local agencies knew about its programs: Agencies knew the outreach worker better than they knew the project, and the outreach worker represented the project to the community.

A second method of outreach was brochures, public service announcements, radio shows, videos, advertising campaigns, and presentations to community agencies. Six of the 10 programs used this method. One program produced its own video, describing the program's various components. However, the program does not recommend using this technique: The video was expensive to produce and it quickly became outdated as the program changed to meet client needs. A popular method of disseminating program information was brochures, which were designed for agencies and were meant to foster referrals. One referral agency thought so highly of a particular brochure that it photocopied it for clients.

Some projects used advertising campaigns and radio shows to reach prospective clients.[27] A program in Detroit designed a poster warning pregnant women of the dangers of using drugs, and placed the poster on city buses. Other programs developed public service announcements.

> *Several of our clients wrote and delivered a script for a public service announcement. The message they conveyed was, "If you are pregnant or just gave birth and using drugs, come to the program we attend for the help you need. It really works." They included the name of the program and the telephone number. It aired on several local radio stations and we documented that new clients called our program to enroll after they heard the broadcast.*
>
> Elizabeth Toledo

Another program had its own call-in talk show on the Spanish radio station.

> *We were targeting Hispanic women for our program and having a difficult time recruiting partly because their families did not want them out of the family environment. Our program director sponsored a program every two weeks to address health concerns of women. She targeted substance abuse whenever she could and included the name and phone number of our project. The fact that this information was coming into people's homes seemed to make treatment more positive for their families, who then supported them coming into treatment.*
>
> Peggy Glider

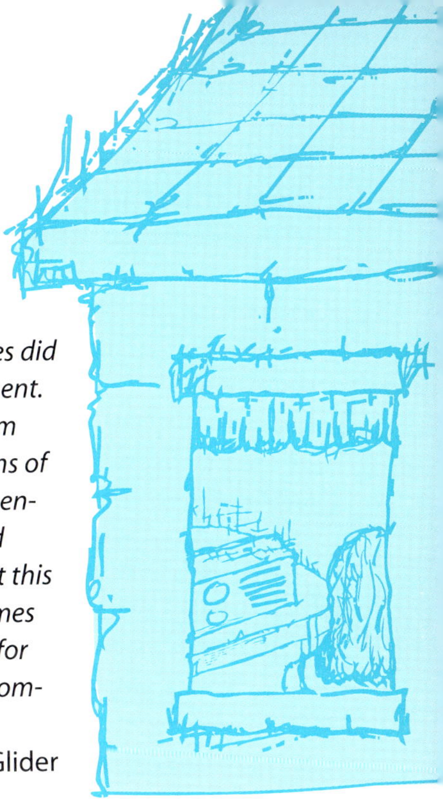

The use of advertising and media approaches for outreach to substance-using pregnant and parenting women is widespread. National and local campaigns against use of tobacco, alcohol, and other drugs during pregnancy are common and have been shown to be effective.[28]

Cultural sensitivity of program and staff: Cultural sensitivity to the ethnic backgrounds of the clients is critical to establishing substance abuse programs as a place where women would want to come. Sometimes, substance-using pregnant women experience poor treatment by professionals who express negative attitudes towards them, believing they should be punished for their addictions. The focus group felt strongly that unless a program communicates understanding and acceptance, recruitment will be difficult. Several specific program characteristics were mentioned.

First, programs must establish a sense of trust and understanding. This may mean that women and their families are told that children will not be removed automatically from the mother. Rather, reunification is promoted whenever possible. To this end, caseworkers and other staff must be seen as advocates. Trust is not easy to establish. Many women require several tries before they are ready to become clients. Often, the first contact with a staff member becomes the strongest link to the program. Staff must be viewed as "nice" and have the philosophy that every addict is ready for help at some level. It is up to the program to identify that level and to meet the client at her level of readiness. Thus staff must be carefully selected and oriented to the importance of the effect of their approach and manner on recruitment. One bad encounter, such as the social worker who tried to convince women to leave their male partners, communicates a lack of understanding of the lifestyles of substance-using women and of their need to move slowly in resolving interpersonal problems.

Several programs discovered that they lost clients early in the enrollment process when staff asked too many questions or probed too deeply into the women's lives. Thus, it was suggested that programs not obtain all the needed information at the first session.

> *I believe that one of the biggest problems we had attracting Latinas was our intake process. When our program first began, we had a very long interview questionnaire that had to be completed on the first day. We noticed that clients would complete the form and never return. We decided that we were asking too much information too early in the client's entry and so we changed our approach. Now, we ask questions over a period of several weeks. This allows us to establish a trusting relationship with our clients before we probe into their private lives. We feel we are able to get more truthful answers in this manner.*
>
> Margery Brooks

Programs also learned that it was important that staff reflect the ethnicity and speak the language of the target population. One program in Hartford targeted Latinas. This was the only program to provide bilingual physicians and other staff—an essential component for group and one-on-one counseling. Several reports document that this may also be critical when using outreach workers, especially in the Hispanic community.[29,30] One report adds that employing same-culture staff also strengthens relationships between the local community and the agency.[30] Other programs that had difficulty recruiting women of a particular ethnic group recognized that lacking staff of that ethnicity played an important part in the difficulty.

A related issue of culture, but not necessarily of ethnicity, is the importance of project staff understanding the language, values, and lifestyles of the clients. Many programs employed recovering addicts as caseworkers and outreach workers to bridge an understanding between the project and its clients. Other successful projects have found that recovering addicts who are on staff speak the same language as the clients and are better able to access recruitment networks. Some staff continue to live in the same neighborhoods as their clients.

A second characteristic of cultural sensitivity is for programs to be flexible in meeting client's needs and in working with the existing system of care. As one PPWI group member expressed it, "You have to go to where the women are and that includes the streets. You can't expect them to come to you. You also have to be there when they need you, whether it's for housing or to get their children back."

Substance-using women are often part of an extensive network of other substance users. For example, the program may target a man who may then recruit his pregnant or parenting partner. Alliances with drug dealers were critical to the success of a drug treatment and AIDS program in Puerto Rico.[31] In an ethnographic evaluation, outreach workers detected a sense of caring between dealers and their long-time customers. Additionally, dealers understood that addiction is a chronic condition with many attempts at drug-free living. Many dealers believed that a short "rest" would be "good" for addicts.

Women addicted to drugs live in social environments where there is little long-term planning. Many adapt to their lifestyles by assuming a crisis orientation to decision-making, which may manifest in an inability to wait to access services, including treatment. Therefore, substance abuse treatment providers must reduce the waiting time from the initial contact to entry into the program. Most of the programs represented in the focus group admitted clients immediately, or within a few days. When programs were full, staff attempted to maintain contact with prospective clients.

Flexibility was also seen as important in working with a changing system of care. For example, when managed care providers began recruiting pregnant women on Medicaid in large numbers, several projects found it necessary to alter their referral patterns and establish contracts with HMOs to screen and/or provide treatment for their clients. This was often difficult, as most managed care providers were reluctant to support treatment programs that were longer than 60 to 90 days.

Programs must be flexible in their appointment structure. Substance-users' lifestyles are not organized around an appointment schedule that requires that they wait a week, or even several days, before entering the program. As one project director stated, "They are not thinking six months down the road. They think in the short term, and so must we."

Placing emphasis on the responsibility of the mother towards her unborn/newborn often made women feel valued. Since being pregnant was often the incentive for women to begin treatment, programs stressed the importance of reducing or eliminating drugs for the infants' health. This unique feature of PPWI programs brought in pregnant women when other substance abuse programs failed to recruit these women.

Providing special services, such as child care, may be essential to a recruitment effort.

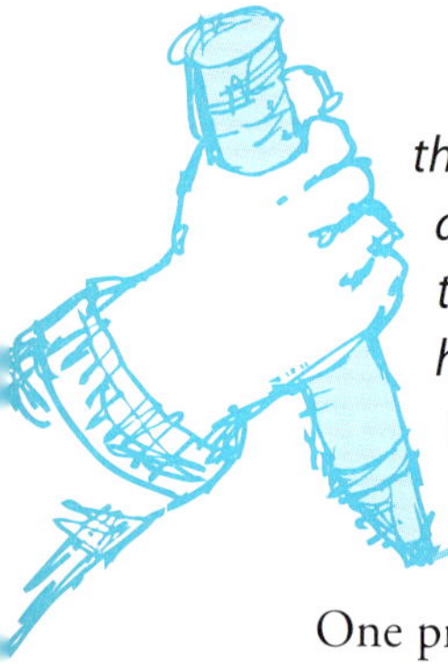

Intensive day care is rare in our city. We provided a therapeutic learning center for our children from birth to age five years. Our clients spend time in the center with their children, having lunch there and participating in hands-on activities. Child Protective Service liked to refer to us because they knew we had the learning center.

Peggy Glider

One program found that its spirituality component attracted women who felt that it addressed an important unmet need.

We hired a new counselor who was interested in working with the women and their issues related to spirituality. She started a spirituality group that was very popular. We noted that women would miss one-on-one sessions with other counselors, but would not miss the spirituality sessions. Our program became widely known for offering this service and several of the clients who completed our program mentioned to me that the spirituality sessions helped to make them mentally ready to begin the hard work of recovery.

Margery Brooks

Another program realized that many substance-using women had an unmet need for laundry facilities. The program felt that if it made these facilities available to all female addicts, they would be attracted to the program. The program placed two washers and two dryers in the center's basement and opened it to their clients and to any nonclient substance-using woman. The laundry was open from 7:00 a.m. until 7:30 p.m. and provided a needed service, as well as a safe place for the women to congregate. Over time, the program recruited women who were initially reluctant to seek treatment.

Incentives: Although offering incentives is popular in substance abuse treatment programs, there is no evidence that this approach is effective in recruiting and retaining clients.[3,27] In 1986, the Institute of Medicine convened the interdisciplinary Committee to Study Outreach for Prenatal Care to examine ways of drawing more women into prenatal care early in pregnancy.[32] The committee found little evidence that either case or in-kind incentives brought women into care, although data in this area are extremely limited.

Six programs offered incentives of monetary value. Most programs collected clothing and baby items to have available as incentives for their clients to remain in the program. However, one project conducted community baby showers to recruit women into prenatal care and, indirectly, into its program. The use of incentives did not appear to be a successful recruitment strategy.

> *We organized large community baby showers as one way to recruit unregistered women into prenatal care and, subsequently, into our program. The showers were held in churches and other community facilities. Clothing, toiletries, baby items, and other gifts were donated for the women and infants who attended. Public health nurses screened women for blood pressure and for enrollment in prenatal and infant care services. Classes were held on nutrition, child care, parenting, and other subjects. Although the showers were well attended, they were not effective in recruiting nonregistered pregnant women or women using substances.*
>
> Lisa Potti

Another project sponsored a health fair, with educational and play activities for families with young children. As with the baby showers, few families were found that were not already enrolled in health care. Drug screening was not seen as an appropriate activity for a health fair.

One incentive thought to be effective is the drug-free "dollars" program.

> *We offer drug-free dollars to our clients for submitting urine screens and complying with offered services. For example, women receive a dollar for intake, for drug screening, and for lab work. For each month of clean urine toxicologies, the client receives five dollars. If the client delivers a drug-free baby, she receives 10 dollars. These dollars are really certificates that can be traded in for items in our catalog. Staff and clients selected items they thought would be appropriate.*
>
> *Although we have no concrete evidence that this incentive is effective in recruiting clients, the program is very popular. We found, for example, that clients who need to have two lab tests will have one on Friday and return on Monday for the second, instead of having both on the same day. This earns them two drug-free dollars instead of one.*
>
> Susan Cox

Barriers to Recruitment

The focus group listed many barriers to recruiting pregnant substance-using women, including racial stereotyping, negative attitudes towards substance-users, insurance problems, cultural beliefs and practices, lack of family and/or partner support, and the general structure and philosophy of programs.

Stereotyping: Health professionals often believed that women who used drugs were exclusively low income and African American. Caucasian, Hispanic, and Asian women were often overlooked and were screened less often than African-American women because "they don't use drugs." Women who dressed well were also viewed as "too nice" to use drugs. Projects noted that, at times, outreach strategies such as distributing pamphlets and television advertisements focused on low-income women and reinforced stereotypes. All of the participants shared examples of these stereotypes and agreed that to overcome them training of professionals was critical.

Negative attitudes: General negative attitudes of professionals towards women who use drugs, especially pregnant women, were seen in prenatal clinics refusing to screen or care for substance-using women and in drug treatment programs that would not treat pregnant women. Some of the bias was due to the belief that "those women are all high risk," and some agencies felt unprepared or unwilling to care for them. There was also the perception that substance-using women were more likely to sue for medical malpractice and were upsetting to nonusers if both were seen in the same setting.

Insurance problems: Insurance problems presented another major barrier to recruitment into substance abuse programs. Problems included insurance companies that would not cover the costs of long-term treatment and managed care contracts that provided their own in-house treatment.

> *We had a client who worked at a local department store full time. She wanted to enter our treatment program, but her insurance refused to cover the costs. Instead, they referred her to a four-week program that would not take her because she was pregnant. She finally quit her job and qualified for Medicaid and disability. Then we could take her. The problem now is that she has delivered, and she qualifies for only 90 days of treatment. It takes us about 90 days of treatment just to clear the fog. Then we can begin serious treatment.*
>
> Susan Cox

Managed care: Managed care presents problems to most programs, often resulting in sudden changes in coverage for a client already in treatment. Several projects described prospective pregnant clients who were ready to enter the programs but suddenly found themselves enrolled in a health maintenance organization (HMO) that would not allow them to seek treatment at the PPWI sites. This often happened to large numbers of prospective clients when states mandated managed care and all pregnant women had to enroll in managed care clinics. Additionally, old referral patterns were disrupted and the new managed care providers either did not screen for substance use or developed their own in-house treatment. Several PPWI programs had to alter recruitment strategies to find new sources of potential clients; a few worked with managed care providers to continue to serve this population.

Cultural differences: Culturally prescribed norms often dictated whether or not it was proper for a woman to admit to substance use, to answer questions about use within her family, or to seek help. These norms affected recruitment. Two projects found that pregnant Hispanic women were most likely to underreport substance use. Additionally, questions about family substance use were often seen as invading the family's privacy; this information would not be divulged until women had been in the program for several months. The programs also felt that many Hispanic families believed that substance use problems must remain, and were best dealt with, in the family. Latinas did not take their problems, especially those that reflected larger family issues, to strangers. Pregnancy magnified all of these cultural barriers, since drug use during pregnancy added an additional stigma.

Lack of family/partner support: Another barrier to recruiting pregnant women was lack of support from family and male partners. Some families did not want the woman to admit to outsiders, including program staff, that she was using drugs. There was concern that private family matters would be shared with strangers. Male partners who continued to use drugs were particularly controlling, often sabotaging outreach and other recruitment efforts. The women were generally protective of their male partners and several programs learned that it was important to address the male partners' needs before they would allow the women to enter treatment.

Program structure: Programs that were not structured to meet the needs of specific ethnic or socioeconomic groups were unable to recruit these women. For example, not having bilingual staff was a barrier to recruiting women who spoke Spanish. Having a primarily unicultural staff discouraged a multicultural clientele. One program, with a local population of 14 percent Native American women and no Native American staff, suspected that their low recruitment of 1.9 percent Native American client population was due, in part, to lack of Native American staff.

Programs that targeted low-income women found that they did not attract middle-income women. In fact, few PPWI programs attracted middle-income women. One proposed reason was that private physicians serving middle-income women were less likely to screen their patients for substance use than those serving low-income women. Few programs had any success recruiting adolescents because program materials and foci were primarily on adult women.

Lessons Learned

1. Substance-using pregnant women are generally difficult to recruit into a variety of health and social service programs including drug treatment programs.
2. To be successful at recruitment, programs must be flexible in their approaches and use a variety of recruitment strategies. This may include outreach to families and male partners as well as recruiting women in places where they spend time.
3. Pregnant women who use substances represent a unique, but diverse, group of women with special psychosocial needs and lifestyles. Their lifestyles must be understood and their needs addressed in order to recruit them into needed services. They often have a fear of health professionals and law enforcement.
4. Recruitment efforts will vary depending on the role of a program within the established system of care. Programs should establish a niche within the system of care and identify several approaches to recruitment to maximize their successes.
5. Cultural beliefs and attitudes play an important role in how women and their families feel about substance use and treatment. Programs have to take this into account in staffing their programs and addressing culturally prescribed norms.
6. Substance abuse programs must become involved in ongoing training of professionals in other agencies in techniques related to screening and referral, and to help them overcome biases regarding pregnant women who use substances.
7. Hiring paraprofessionals and/or recovering persons enhances recruitment efforts through modeling to clients that recovery is possible. It also helps nonrecovering staff better understand the addiction process. ■

Chapter 3

Retention

Lack of retention of substance-using pregnant and parenting women in a variety of health and social service programs, including drug treatment, has been described as a barrier to the successful completion of a variety of services set up for this population. Additionally, the concept of retention has been difficult for programs to define and measure.

Substance use, including addiction, is a chronic relapsing condition often requiring long-term treatment. For many addicts, there are multiple starting and ending periods, as they begin and terminate drug treatment for a variety of reasons.

The PPWI focus group defined retention as "a goal-directed activity designed to keep clients and families engaged in services in order to attain outcomes mutually agreed upon by the client and staff." While all group participants supported this definition, its application to their programs and the manner in which retention was measured varied.

Measurement of retention was difficult for several reasons. Some clients attended the program for a period of time without any real commitment to changing their lifestyles or drug use, or they dropped out and then returned. There were discussions regarding at what point women actually became clients, raising questions about how to measure both the beginning and the ending of services and involvement in programs. Some clients had vague endpoints—they reached their treatment goals, but returned or were monitored periodically for relapse prevention. Those programs with clearly established endpoints had difficulty maintaining them. For example, some clients who were close to reaching an established endpoint became pregnant again. All programs continued to follow these clients, thus prolonging their time in the program.

Residential drug treatment programs have obvious endpoints particularly when the client physically leaves the program. However, intensive day treatment or other kinds of outpatient programs are generally recommended after the client leaves residential treatment. And this latter involvement is more difficult to measure. Thus, absolute, quantifiable beginning and ending periods are difficult to measure, and make retention a problematic area of study.

Types of Retention

Focus group members described three specific types of retention: (1) goal directed, (2) time limited, and (3) mixed. Goal directed was defined as having the clients and staff establish agreed-upon goals and treatment plans, such as a decrease in drug use or the delivery of a drug-free infant. Four programs used goal-directed endpoints for length of retention. When clients reached these goals, they were usually discharged from the program. Some programs responded to the needs and motivation of the client and did not push her into a treatment that she did not want or was not ready for at the time. For instance, delivering a drug-free infant concentrated on the short-term goal of decreasing substance use during pregnancy, instead of focusing on long-term recovery. There were instances when staff felt clients had attained their goals, but clients felt they were not ready to leave the program. In these situations, programs often retained clients until they felt ready to leave the program.

Three programs established time-limited endpoints for retention, such as one to three years after delivery. Case managers worked with clients to reach goals during this period, reducing the intensity of contact over time. All three time-limited programs identified instances where clients were retained in the program past the endpoint or returned to the program after discharge.

Three programs described a mixed approach to retention using established treatment goals and time-limited periods. These programs worked towards treatment goals over an agreed-upon time period, but clients often remained in the program for many years (due in one case to the placement of the program in a primary care center and, in another case, to instituting long-term followup for relapse prevention). One of these programs discharged clients when there was no contact after 60 days, although they readmitted several of these discharged clients. Another program advised its clients to return when they felt they were having a relapse.

There are few data on why women (or men) remain in treatment or drop out before a therapeutic goal is achieved. Some of the factors associated with short-stay retention include low motivation for long-term abstinence, dual diagnosis, lack of support from families and male partners, low educational level, and concern over family responsibilities such as caring for young children.[33,34]

Median lengths of stay for men have been shown to be similar to those of women in residential and outpatient substance abuse treatment programs when programs address issues such as family responsibilities and transportation.[35–37] Programs that offer more services, including residential treatment, generally experience longer retention. Shorter lengths of stay have also been associated with cocaine use, younger age, use of multiple substances, and social isolation.[38] Reports on the effect of involvement in the criminal justice system differ.[38,39] A study by Collins and Allison found that clients who are referred to drug treatment by legal means are more likely to remain in treatment longer than those not mandated.[39] Further, mandated clients are just as likely as nonmandated clients to reach their therapeutic goals.

Median lengths of stay vary widely across programs, from 35 days to 18 months.[40,41] Studies on the impact of treatment length support that longer retention is associated with lower rates of substance use, criminal behavior, and unemployment.[34,42] However, less than half of the clients in many programs remain in treatment for three months, which is the minimum time considered necessary for a therapeutic effect.[43] Some may seek short-term treatment as a "drug holiday" from the physical effects of and the lifestyle associated with drug use, instead of seeking long-term recovery.[44]

Thus, measuring retention in a drug treatment program presents a dilemma: When exactly does drug treatment begin, and when does it end? The answers may be different for the program versus the client, and for many clients treatment involves several beginnings and endings. Since the focus group members could not arrive at a satisfactory measurement, they agreed that retention began when the client received some kind of assessment and participated in project activities, and ended when the client was formally discharged from the program.

Retention Strategies

The 10 group participants listed many strategies they used to retain clients. These strategies may be classified into three general categories: physical environment and approach, removing barriers, and special incentives.

Physical environment and approach: The first area discussed under physical environment and approach was the resources available to clients. Several participants mentioned that the program had to look welcoming; this meant appropriate pictures and comfortable chairs for group settings. This area, by far, elicited the most discussion.

One program tried to make itself homelike, so women would feel comfortable and safe. Clients were engaged in designing and decorating the center; some brought pictures and other items from home. Pictures of former clients were displayed in the same way photos of family members are displayed in a home. Clients were also encouraged to write welcoming letters, describing their experiences in the center, for new clients. When a new client entered the program, she was given a book of letters to read. Comfort was also important. Program staff did not want clients sitting on hard chairs during group sessions, so they purchased overstuffed chairs.

Arrangements for child care, especially that which could be offered on-site, was another important component that added to the homelike atmosphere. Several programs offered food on-site, including having clients participate in meal preparation. Serving food was also incorporated into parenting since mothers prepared food and served it to their young children. Staff participated in these meals, modeling healthy family behavior and the importance of families gathering together at mealtime.

Having sufficient physical space to create private areas was also critical.

> *We had a problem in our prenatal clinic in that there was no privacy for confidential discussions of substance use, sexual abuse, and other sensitive areas of the clients' lives. We were also concerned about protecting confidential written information that was included in clients' charts.*

We established private offices, away from the busy area of the prenatal care clinic. Here, women could feel comfortable enough to disclose very personal information. We were also careful to protect this information in the medical chart. We maintained two charts on each client. One was the medical record in which we recorded answers to screening questions; the second contained more detailed notes from the social worker's interview with the client. While both charts were kept in locked cabinets, the second chart was stored in the private offices, away from the rest of the clinic charts. Establishing private areas and protecting sensitive information fostered the client's trust and improved staff-client relationships.

Sally Carter

A second retention strategy, closely aligned to the first, was establishing a "feeling tone" within the project that encouraged clients to bring their problems to the staff. Several projects learned to establish this feeling tone early for clients by not asking very personal and difficult questions until the relationship was well established. Thus, questions about history of sexual and physical abuse were often discussed after the client had been in the program for weeks or months. Trust in the program staff was also established by clearly stating program rules. Clients did not complain about urine toxicology screens when they knew that they would be conducted and the reason for them.

Two things that disrupted a healthy feeling tone for clients were the loss of case management staff and staff having caseloads that were too large. Clients often dropped out of the program when a trusted case manager left. Discontinuity of case management, especially when clients were not followed by a team, was often described by clients as similar to losing a close friend. A different problem occurred when clients were retained and new clients were added to existing caseloads. It was believed that case managers with caseloads as high as 80 clients no longer had time to give personal attention to their clients. The feeling tone of the program suffered and management had to make decisions either to add new staff or discharge clients.

Many clients had never previously experienced a healthy family lifestyle and found for the first time, in the treatment center, what it meant to feel cared for. The treatment environment, including how clients perceive staff caring for them, has a major effect on retention.[45] In PPWI programs the treatment staff and clients became the client's family, at least temporarily. This was seen most vividly for one project when a client requested that the project staff help her with her wedding. She had always dreamed of a large wedding, but her family and friends, most of whom were drug addicted, were not stable enough to assist in the planning. Program staff and clients became involved in the wedding. The wedding gown was designed and made by staff and clients; food was prepared by the clients, and the hospital chaplain conducted the service. At the last minute, the maid of honor failed to appear (she was on the streets getting high) and the project director stepped in to fill that role. The wedding was described by the client as "a dream come true" and many of the other clients experienced, firsthand, how healthy families support members during special events.

Several projects agreed that for substance-using women who had grown up in families where drugs often interfered with celebrating special milestones, the family atmosphere of the treatment center modeled healthy relationships and established newfound family traditions. Client birthdays and their children's birthdays were often celebrated. Clients connected with each other by sharing these milestones. One program director continues to receive invitations to parties from former clients even though the program has ended.

In addition to parties, the special feeling tone established by the project included helping women learn to support each other in dealing with difficult issues. According to one study, support from staff and "sister" clients was a powerful incentive to completing treatment.[46] One program organized retreats (the clients called them slumber parties), for 24 to 48 hours of intensive work. Sensitive topics were dealt with that could not be expressed or handled in ambulatory settings. Another project had all-day rap sessions that were organized by the clients. This fostered organization and planning and gave women a sense of pride and ownership in their treatment.

Many clients referred to the treatment program staff as "the only real family I have." The family atmosphere was not only part of the treatment, but helped retain many women. According to one focus group participant, "that is what is really unique about the work that we do." Other published reports support this statement.[46]

The third area under physical environment is client input into treatment programs. This was described earlier as it related to clients creating a homelike atmosphere. But several programs took this a step further by periodically conducting focus group discussions with clients to elicit suggestions for program change. Five programs hired their own graduates to foster client perspective into treatment.

> *We conducted focus group discussions once a year to ask clients how we could make our program better. One request they made was for someone to be available at night, for relapse and child-abuse prevention counseling. We wrote a grant and obtained funding for a parent aide to be available in the evenings, after our staff had left. We hired and trained a paraprofessional for this position. The person we hired was a former client. This sent a message to our other clients that we not only listened to them and acted upon their advice, but we were even able to hire one of them. This parent aide is sensitive to the needs of the clients because she has been there herself. This further reinforces our respect for the expertise of our clients.*
>
> *The client we hired had been receiving Aid to Families with Dependent Children. She is now supporting herself and her child. This is a powerful message to other women that economic self-sufficiency is possible.*
>
> Elizabeth Toledo

Other projects used focus groups in a similar way. One project moved to a different location on the advice of clients. Another used the focus group discussions as an opportunity to find clients who had dropped out of the program. Former clients were invited back to participate in the group discussion surrounding improvements needed in the program. Former clients were often re-recruited in this manner. Several program participants pointed out that program changes often present difficult adjustments for clients. Therefore, including clients in the decision to change components of the program helps ease the adjustment and promotes buy-in on the part of clients.

Five of the 10 programs hired former clients as paraprofessionals and peer counselors. All felt that this gave an important message to current clients regarding their abilities to become employed and that their experiences as recovering addicts were invaluable to the program. One program that needed peer counselors but had no funds to pay a salary rewarded clients with coupons for food and other items in exchange for their acting as peer counselors. The experience was important to the women and helped them gain future employment.

The fourth area under physical environment and approach addresses the nature of support received from the staff. Creating an emotionally safe and supportive environment for women in treatment allows issues of sexual, physical, and emotional abuse to be addressed at a rate appropriate for each individual.[47] Providing resources, such as child care and transportation, certainly helped women remain in the program, but assistance in less tangible forms was also mentioned. Substance-using women often lack stable social supports and survive on a day-to-day basis.[48] One program noted that difficulty finding suitable housing kept clients from being retained in their programs. Therefore, they hired a housing specialist to assist clients obtain safe, affordable housing.

Another program, realizing that it was not enough for clients to come to the program, added home visiting to its retention strategies. This helped staff maintain contact with clients on a regular basis and reminded clients that staff cared about them when they were not at the treatment center. One project used a buddy system to find out why clients missed appointments. Each client was matched with a buddy; if the client missed an appointment, the buddy was responsible for contacting her to find out if she or the program staff could be of assistance. Another program had a policy of identifying a friendly neighbor or, more importantly, the client's mother. These individuals were notified when clients failed appointments and they were often successful in encouraging clients to remain in the program. These activities also reminded clients that their participation in treatment was important to the staff and fellow clients.

Staff attitudes towards treatment also influenced treatment outcomes. One project, part of a large primary care setting, noted that attitudes of nurses, physicians, ultrasound technicians, registration clerks, and all others in the system affected how clients felt about their treatment. Therefore, the project oriented all staff to the importance of staff attitudes about retention of substance-using women. Additionally, fostering trust in staff by maintaining client anonymity whenever possible aids retention.[49]

Advocacy was mentioned by several programs as an important retention strategy. Advocacy occurred at both an individual and a community level. Individual advocacy occurred when clients needed support in court or in regaining custody of their children. Often, clients lacked the education and self-confidence to speak effectively for themselves. Caseworkers accompanied clients and provided the moral support and practical guides necessary for them to negotiate with a child protection worker or the courts. Clients who remained involved with programs learned that staff would remain involved with them and their problems. This was an incentive to continue participation. Clients became empowered as they learned to speak for themselves and their children.

Community advocacy encouraged clients to become involved with legislation related to substance abuse, to convince elected officials of the need for additional services, and to support similar groups wanting change. One program paid for child care and transportation so clients could testify before their state legislature regarding the need for a new treatment center for women and their children. Clients used their own experiences to illustrate the need for this service and they were successful in persuading elected officials to open a new treatment center for this purpose. Clients felt, for the first time, that they could have a powerful impact. The involvement in this kind of advocacy kept women in treatment by demonstrating that their knowledge and experiences were valuable and that, by learning how to organize their efforts, they could succeed.

Another program advocated on behalf of maternity services.

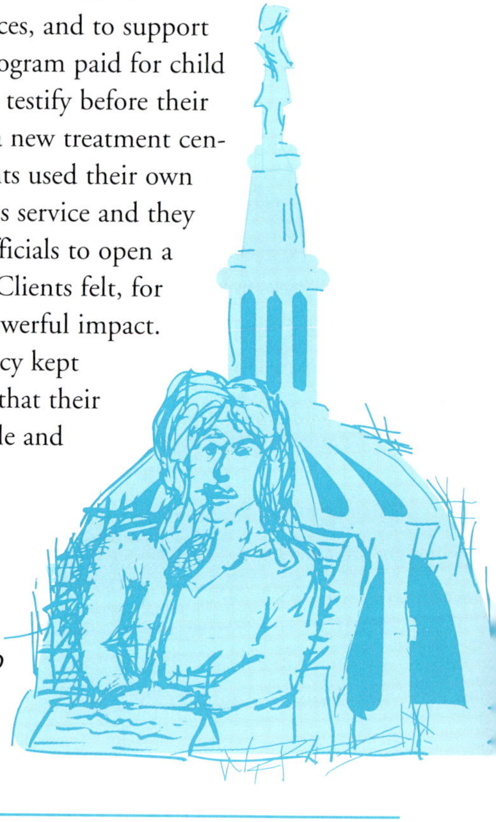

Our state legislature wanted to reduce funding for maternity and substance abuse services. Several

of our clients volunteered to testify before the legislature and they were successful in preventing budget cuts. The knowledge that they could change legislation empowered them. The fact that the program staff actively supported this effort communicated to them that we saw ourselves as a team, working together, to improve conditions for women and children.

Elizabeth Toledo

The fifth retention strategy used in physical environment and approach involved the nature of the treatment itself, including gender and cultural sensitivity, comprehensive approaches to addressing women's needs, and spirituality. Providing gender-specific and culturally sensitive services was viewed as critical to retaining women, especially minority women. Programs that were the most successful at this hired staff from cultures reflecting their client population. Two programs hired male caseworkers to help women develop healthy relationships with men.

Gender-specific services were seen as important in child care, reproductive, and pediatric health care services that were provided. The sensitive manner in which the gender-specific treatment was provided also aided retention. Length of stay for women in treatment can be increased when gender-specific programming is introduced.[50] The only male member of the focus group expressed it this way:

I have been involved in both all male and all female substance abuse programs. Men are able to focus on themselves in treatment. Women have "baggage" that men do not have to deal with. Women, especially pregnant and parenting women, are under social pressure to parent their children. They are often made to feel that they failed if they use drugs and they are made to feel bad about themselves. Therefore, three things are critical for treatment programs to do for women if they are to succeed in treatment: Address their low self-esteem, model nurturing behavior, and help them establish healthy relationships with others, especially with healthy men.

Stephen Ridley

Male caseworkers have special roles to play in women's drug treatment programs. First, men may be uniquely suited to work with male partners who are reluctant to become involved in the women's treatment. However, they must first establish themselves as caseworkers, not as competitors to the male partner. Second, male caseworkers may provide the first healthy relationship that some female clients establish with a man. This is important to explore with female clients, as male caseworkers tend to model healthy relationships.

Group participants felt strongly that substance-using women are treated differently than are substance-using men. Punitive state laws punish women who use drugs, including alcohol, during pregnancy. Media attention reminds women of the special pressures on them not to use substances. On the other hand, men who kill pedestrians while driving drunk receive less press attention. These differences leave lasting impressions on substance-using women that treatment programs must address. At times, women are made to feel more guilty than men about their substance use and this, along with frequent histories of physical and sexual abuse, may be associated with higher rates of depression in women. According to a 1980 National Institute on Drug Abuse (NIDA) study, 70 percent of addicted women reported that they had been raped or physically abused prior to their substance use.[51]

Another gender-specific difference that may affect retention involves the very basic way that women view their social environments. Men generally define themselves through their work. Women often define themselves through their relationships with others.[52] Substance-using women are likely to have been introduced to drugs through their male partners.[6] In a large study of women in a drug treatment program, only 13 percent of Caucasian women and 16 percent of African-American women had partners who were not abusing drugs.[53] In a case-controlled study of 237 pregnant women, 74 percent of drug users had a family history of alcohol or drug problems while 44 percent of nonusers had a family history of substance use.[6] Since family history of substance use and having a male partner who uses substances strongly influence whether women use drugs during pregnancy, interventions should address pregnant women in the context of their family and male relationships, and be sensitive to the environments these women come from and will likely return to following drug treatment. On the one hand, relationships that women establish with substance-using men are important to their definitions of themselves. On the other hand, learning to establish relationships with healthy men is important to long-term recovery.

Substance abuse programs for women must understand this dilemma and address relationships in ways that do not unduly threaten women (and their substance-using male partners), causing them to leave treatment before completion. One program attempted to overcome this dilemma by maintaining contact with current and former clients through a newsletter. The newsletter contained information about relationships and other gender-specific topics that promoted healthy relationships with family, friends, children, and male partners. Other programs used recovering women to speak to those still using substances to address the need to establish healthy relationships. These women acted as role models to clients attempting to alter their relationships with men.

Another aspect of helping clients in treatment establish relationships was working with them to confront others in a healthy manner. Traditional drug treatment programs frequently use an aggressively confrontational approach with clients designed to break through denial. Relapse evokes a punitive response rather than exploration of environmental factors related to resuming drug use. Treatment approaches recommended for women include confronting the behavior—not the individual. This approach maintains relationships among participants; women often appear more comfortable with this approach.

Integrating cultural beliefs and practices into programs helped minority women feel more at home and understood by treatment staff. One program, which addressed the needs of Latinas, discovered that they had to become more sensitive to the different needs and perspectives of Dominican versus Puerto Rican women. This required staff training. Still, according to one report, Hispanic women are more difficult to retain in substance abuse treatment programs than Caucasian women or women of other minority groups.[54]

All programs celebrated ethnic holidays and traditions. Those who served Latinas hired bilingual staff and translated forms and informational materials into Spanish. But beyond the need to be sensitive to language and customs was the need to address what one program described as "oppression illness" (Elizabeth Toledo). They recognized that loss of self-esteem due to socialization into the female role was magnified by the additional stresses of coping with racism: "You cannot begin to touch the issue of self-esteem in women of color until you help them deal with the internalized residue of institutionalized sexism and racism."

This program adapted Mujeres Anonimas: Women Anonymous/Cuidate Mujer: Twelve Steps Model for Latina Women.

> *Based on the 12-step model, the group has been adapted to the cultural, social, and linguistic needs of Latina women. The group is open to all Latina women in the Hartford community. Some of the adaptations include:*
>
> - *Respeto: Respect for themselves and each other*
> - *Responsabilidad Communal: Shared responsibility for the community*
> - *Confianza: Goes beyond trust to feelings of comfort and ease*
> - *Combating sexism and racism in ourselves and in others*
> - *Spirituality is more prominent than a higher power, with no mention of any organized religion or deity.*
>
> *The group operates under strict rules regarding anonymity, proper words, topics, and behavior, and no use of drugs. Members who remain clean are recognized with key tags at 30, 60, and 90 days; 6, 9, and 12 months.*
>
> Elizabeth Toledo

Finally, two specific aspects of the program also helped retain women in treatment: (1) introducing the topic of spirituality into group sessions, and (2) integrating treatment into comprehensive primary care. Participants had difficulty defining spirituality, but they all agreed on particular applications it had for drug treatment. Discussions about spirituality frequently connected women to something they lost—e.g., their cultures, themselves, or their relationships with others or higher beings. Many clients were uncomfortable with religion, but could connect with, as one program described the spirituality component, "working on our inner selves." Programs introduced Native American spirituality, affirmations, yoga, and meditation. One program found a volunteer to introduce the clients to drumming as the group discussed women's journeys through life.

The kind of support that programs provided extended into comprehensive care. Integrating drug treatment into comprehensive health and social services through case management helped retain clients in the program and ease women back into the community.

We hired a case manager to coordinate our clients' care among other agencies. The case manager would contact all of the staff from agencies involved in a particular case to ensure continuum of care. Often, clients were invited to these multidisciplinary staff meetings to make sure the client agreed to the coordinated plan. We also had a regular tracking system for all of our high-risk patients. Whenever a patient missed an appointment, we made contact with her by phone or by home visit. These approaches helped maintain women in our program and in the other programs as well.

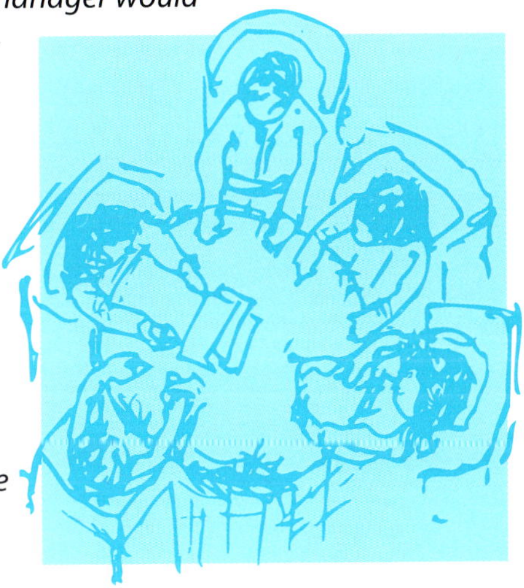

Sally Carter

A program in Detroit that evaluated the effectiveness of its case management approach found that it contributed significantly to retention in drug treatment.[55] The program also reported that providing transportation to drug treatment and prenatal care enhanced retention.

Providing comprehensive services in one location improved retention. Several projects were connected to primary care or other health care providers. Linking women with mental health and reproductive services, along with providing nutrition, parenting, and HIV prevention education helps to retain women in all of these services. Participants stressed that having services in one place increased access to all services, while referring women to places outside of the immediate system often failed due to lack of transportation and child care as well as lack of motivation to seek services in unfamiliar settings.

Removing barriers to retention: Group participants referred to several barriers to retention in substance abuse treatment. First, lack of transportation to treatment and child care presented significant barriers. Nine out of the 10 programs provided free transportation to drug treatment appointments. One of the programs, Mother Infant Substance Abuse Network (MISAN), provided free transportation to substance abuse treatment appointments and to prenatal care. This project's evaluation reported that providing transportation had a statistically significant effect on retention in drug treatment.[55] Eight programs included child care as part of ongoing treatment. This not only eliminated the barrier imposed by lack of child care, but it also introduced the opportunity for the program to teach and reinforce parenting as part of treatment.

Second, clients needed basic necessities before they could continue in treatment. One program experienced a sudden loss of clients when the state welfare agency changed its policy with little warning.

> *Our governor decided that all "able-bodied" adults should be able to find employment. Therefore, with little notice, he discontinued the state's General Assistance program. Several of our clients received General Assistance and used the income for basic necessities such as housing and food. When the assistance was eliminated, they dropped out of treatment and returned to the streets to earn income. Many returned to substance use. We were never able to find most of these women, even though more than half were pregnant at the time.*
>
> Lisa Potti

Finding safe, affordable housing was another ongoing need of clients in all of the projects, and this affected retention. Studies of retention of substance-using women in research projects refer to frequent moves as a major problem.[16] As mentioned earlier, one program hired a housing specialist to address this problem, while others used project social workers to help clients find housing.

Many of the most difficult clients to retain were homeless. As one program director asked, "How can I ask women to commit to five days of outpatient treatment when they don't know where they are going to be sleeping tonight or what school their children will be attending tomorrow?" Stabilizing their lives, including providing safe housing, was necessary before women could commit to remaining in treatment.

Finding health care for acute and ongoing health problems presented a barrier to retention. Nine of the 10 programs found it necessary to provide reproductive health care along with drug treatment and to include pediatric care in the system of care.

Third, clients' families and male partners, especially those who continued to use drugs, often presented barriers to retention. One study found that family involvement significantly increased retention and that programs should involve families to help retain clients.[16,56] Families sometimes pressured women to leave drug treatment programs, especially when family dynamics were disrupted by a change in the client's behavior towards recovery. Some male partners were similarly threatened. Programs discovered the importance of including families and male partners in treatment by offering them group counseling or individual therapy. This helped teach families and male partners the importance of supporting women to remain in treatment.

Women with children with chronic illnesses often stayed away from treatment, because there may have been no one else to care for their children. Additionally, women with several children often needed to supervise them during school breaks and for minor illnesses. One study of the correlates of retention in outpatient treatment found that the more children a mother had, the less likely she was to remain in treatment due to problems with child care.[46] Few programs were able to overcome this barrier.

Fourth, clients with dual diagnosis, especially those with psychosis, were difficult to retain. Most programs did not have the psychiatric support for these women, and their behavior was often disruptive to the other clients. Thus, lack of a psychiatric component to a program presented a barrier to the dually diagnosed.

Incentives: All programs provided incentives, in one form or another, to encourage or reward women for changing their behaviors. This practice is common in substance abuse treatment and research studies of addicts.[48,57] Incentives were usually in the form of gifts and celebrations.

Six of the 10 programs used gifts to reward behavior change or to locate clients who had dropped out of the program. These gifts were donated; no programs had line items in their budgets for incentives.

A quilting club adopted our program. It was their wish that we give homemade quilts to our clients with the name of the quilter in the right-hand corner. They asked that clients write them thank-you notes so that they would be sure that clients received the blankets.

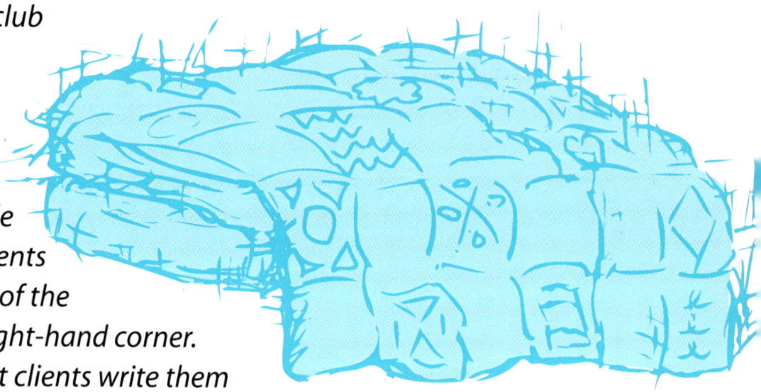

We used the blankets to encourage clients to return to our program. Whenever a client did not attend the program for a period of time, one of our case managers would visit her at home and bring a blanket. This usually helped us gain entry into the home. Most former clients were delighted to receive this beautiful homemade quilt. Then we would explain that she needed to write a thank-you note. We used the thank-you note as a screen for our client's literacy and to send to the woman who quilted the blanket.

Lisa Potti

Other programs were adopted by organizations such as the local police district, schools, clubs, and retirement communities. Most of the gifts came from organizations during Christmas. Two programs noted that neonatal care unit nurses were among the most generous donors to their programs.

Programs received layettes, cribs, baby clothes, toys, and personal items for mothers. These were often presented to clients who were active in the program at the time of delivery to encourage them to remain in the program, because programs felt that this was the time when women were most likely to drop out.

Providing incentives as a reward for a behavior change, including being retained in the program for a specified period of time, was used by eight projects. One program presented clients with gift certificates at three and six months of pregnancy, at delivery, at six months postpartum, and again at graduation from the program. A similar method of using incentives included rewarding clients with a small gift when they completed each of the program's five phases. Another program paid for clients' hair or nail care as a reward for remaining in the program. A fourth program had a small store with items for mothers and children. Clients would obtain coupons for attending group and other activities. They redeemed the coupons for gifts each Friday. Another program instituted a graduated incentive program, providing gift certificates of increasing value to clients who not only completed their program but continued to bring their children back for medical and developmental examinations.

Graduations were used by seven programs to reward clients who completed the program and to encourage those remaining to continue in treatment. Numbers of clients graduating varied from 5 to more than 20. A program in Philadelphia planned elaborate graduations for their clients that were also used as incentives to encourage clients to continue.

> *Our graduations included all of our current and former clients and their families. We instituted a special feature called "clean time countdown." We paired clients with many years of sobriety with those with little time. These pairs gave nonmonetary gifts to each other. For example, a member of the audience with 20 years sobriety would give a gift to a client who had been in our program for two days. This exchange was seen as an acknowledgment of those with many years of sobriety and an incentive for future public acknowledgment to clients recently engaged in treatment.*
>
> Stephen Ridley

One program that received used clothing to distribute to clients and their children found that clients enjoyed returning the clothing when their children outgrew them. Some clients also donated clothing they purchased at garage sales. Donating back to the program acted as an incentive to remain in the program because it represented achievement of stability when clients could now provide for others.

Program staff also donated their clothing to clients. One participant remembered when she mistook a client for a staff member, because the client was wearing a familiar piece of clothing that once belonged to the staff person. Staff helped clients dress for job interviews, and one client once used the staff member's donated used clothing.

Clothing and other resources provided by the community to pregnant and parenting substance-using women not only served as incentives but also forged closer ties between the community and the program. Community groups felt that they were helping individuals and families. Programs had an opportunity to explain their program and the importance of basic necessities to their clients' recovery.

Use of incentives to retain clients in health-related activities is popular across the country; however, there are few studies on their effectiveness. One clinical trial of providing gift certificates for keeping prenatal appointments in a low-income population failed to detect a significant effect.[58] Few patients in this clinical trial were substance users. However, another study involving pregnant substance users found that incentives significantly increased attendance in treatment.[57]

Celebrations represent another kind of incentive that focus group participants believed improved retention. Celebrations were seen as ways to reward clients for achievements or to publicly acknowledge personal milestones. For example, one program sponsored "clean and sober celebrations" for clients whenever they had three months of sobriety. The client celebrating would receive food and presents from clients who had already achieved sobriety or were working towards that goal.

The most elaborate celebrations centered around graduation from the program. Seven programs organized graduations. These usually included a speaker such as the mayor, a health director, or a television personality. Members of the press were often invited. Family and friends of graduating clients were encouraged to attend, as were current clients of the program. Everyone was expected to dress for the occasion and graduates often had their hair done. One focus group member told the story of a graduation celebration at which one graduate was missing: Her hairdo was so elaborate that by the time she completed her coiffure, the ceremony had ended. Certificates were generally given to the graduates, and most were expected to give short speeches about their recoveries and future plans. Graduations were emotional times, especially since most clients "had never graduated from anything before."

The second type of celebration was personal recognition of a milestone or a special holiday. As a participant explained, "Many of our clients never celebrated their own birthdays or learned to celebrate any holiday in a positive way. It is important for staff to model how to celebrate without using drugs." One program sponsored a Mother's Day celebration.

> *Most of our clients were single parents and had never celebrated Mother's Day. We thought their roles as mothers should be rewarded and so we organized a luncheon at an expensive hotel. A local theatrical group performed and a recovering addict read her poetry. Women received gifts and were served an elegant lunch by waiters. Most of the women had never been served like this before and we heard many positive comments about how good the clients felt about this special treatment.*
>
> Lisa Potti

The role of celebrations as a retention strategy is not well described in the literature. However, the group participants felt that the positive reinforcements that came from celebrations and modeling how to have fun without using drugs encouraged clients to remain in the program. Celebrations were also seen as part of the treatment, since they helped to introduce clients into mainstream social and cultural events. There was concern that in the current environment of cost-effectiveness and short-stay, managed care programs, celebrations and other similar strategies would be viewed as superfluous and therefore discontinued. However, the focus group members agreed that celebrations reinforce positive client behavior and should be considered an important retention strategy.

Retention Issues

Group participants summarized retention issues by categorizing clients into two groups; those women who were difficult to retain in programs and those who were easy to retain.

Difficult to retain: Clients who were most difficult to retain in programs tended to be at the extremes of the age range (adolescents and older, hard-core addicts), women with pressure from their families and male partners to leave treatment, women who lacked basic necessities or were mentally ill, and women from cultures different from the staff in the treatment program. Adolescents were difficult to retain because few programs were organized around their special needs. Most clients of drug treatment programs were in their 20s and 30s. Adolescents who participated in drug treatment programs reportedly did not have a peer group with which to interact. When programs are geared to adolescents, their retention rates are comparable to those of adults.[40] Older, hard-core addicts were often less motivated to stop using, especially if they were well integrated into the drug culture. Many sold drugs in addition to using them and were reluctant to give up what in their views were comfortable lifestyles. These were often the clients who used drug treatment as a "holiday" from drugs.

Women were often pressured by family and their male partners to leave treatment for several reasons. First, some families did not want the client in treatment, because they felt that treatment would change her and distance her from the family. Male partners who continued to use substances were particularly difficult to persuade. Second, family responsibilities to care for sick children or supervise children during school vacations kept women out of treatment. One reason clients dropped out of treatment after delivery was that responsibilities for care of a newborn often precluded time for the mother in treatment. The longer clients remained away from treatment, the less likely they were to return. One program instituted an aggressive tracking system to contact clients who missed appointments.

Women who lack housing or who are mentally ill are also difficult to retain. Homeless women have priorities other than treatment and often drop out after a short time. Many are sent to drug treatment by local shelters as a requirement for a bed. Mentally ill women drop out or are referred out because most programs lack the staff to address their special needs.

Finally, clients from ethnic groups different from those of the staff often dropped out because they felt uncomfortable in the treatment setting. Reasons for their discomfort included language barriers and lack of sensitivity to cultural norms. Additionally, since women's programs stress relationships, clients from a different ethnic group may feel isolated from the larger cultural group.

Easy to retain: Clients who were the easiest to retain tended to be self-referred and in early pregnancy, receiving methadone, and having support from family and friends. Women who self-referred were often the most motivated to seek treatment. They tended to enter treatment early in pregnancy and to remain at least through delivery. Many were motivated to reduce or stop substance use because of the pregnancy.

Receiving methadone was another inducement to remain in treatment, at least during pregnancy. Some women transferred from one methadone program to another when they became pregnant, and planned to return to their original program after delivery. However, methadone clients found that PPWI programs were more sensitive to their needs and they tended to remain after delivery, although two program directors felt that methadone clients generally did not mesh well with nonmethadone clients. A study in Detroit found that receiving methadone significantly increased attendance (retention) at an outpatient substance abuse treatment program.

Finally, family and partner support to seek and remain in treatment was essential to retention. Some clients were pressured by their families and male partners to seek treatment when they became pregnant. Several PPWI programs offered counseling to families of clients to help maintain their support of the addicted family member.

Predictors of Retention in Three PPWI Programs

Three participating projects—MISAN, Baybright, and Second Chance—provided data on 551 individual clients to be used in a composite analysis of factors associated with retention (length of stay). The average age of their clients was 27.7 years with a range of 15 to 41; most (69.5 percent) were African American, 18.9 percent were non-Hispanic Caucasian, and 11.4 percent were Hispanic; 98.7 percent were Medicaid eligible. The primary drug of use was cocaine for 64.7 percent of clients; opiates for 19.1 percent. Length of stay (LOS) ranged from 1 to 1,607 days with the mean at 227 days.

Possible predictors of LOS for which projects had comparable data included age, ethnicity, parity, pregnant/not pregnant at the time of recruitment, primary drug of use, and whether or not the admission was court ordered. A correlational analysis identified six factors that were significantly associated with longer LOS: younger age, Caucasian/Hispanic ethnicity, cocaine use, lower parity, nonpregnant, and not court ordered. These factors were entered into a multiple regression analysis with LOS as the criterion (outcome variable). Four factors contributed significantly, explaining 20 percent of the variance for LOS: Caucasian or Hispanic ethnicity, cocaine as the primary drug of choice, not court ordered, and younger age.

This sample cannot be viewed as representative of the 10 projects, and there may be other factors that may explain more of the variance for LOS. Additionally, some of the findings reported here are different from those generally seen in the literature. Those published reports point to older age, court-ordered entry, and primary drug other than cocaine use as factors associated with longer LOS.[38,39] Several reasons are proposed for these differences.

First, the PPWI projects focused on pregnant and parenting women, a group of women who are younger than the general population with pregnancy as a motivation to stop drug use. Court-ordered treatment may have been less effective in this sample when compared with concern for the unborn and fear of child protective services. Second, the PPWI projects were comprehensive, offering many different services. Comprehensive programs generally have longer LOS.[38] Third, the programs were gender specific and designed to be culturally sensitive to their target populations. It may be that when gender-specific programs with a comprehensive array of services are offered to women, the impact of factors such as age, substances used, and mandated treatment on LOS is different. Finally, 64.7 percent of our sample used cocaine as their primary drug. There may not have been sufficient variation in substances used to detect an effect of other substances. Further analyses are necessary before firm conclusions can be drawn.

Lessons Learned

1. Women who are motivated to seek drug treatment often need tangible and emotional support from others to remain in treatment.
2. The physical and social environments of drug treatment programs play an important role in retention. This includes providing a family-like environment where women are comfortable and can find support.
3. Celebrations and other incentives are useful in rewarding behavior change, which also increases retention.
4. Allowing input into the program design empowers clients and improves the treatment approach and retention.

5. Advocacy on behalf of clients models how clients can negotiate with agencies and institutions and further strengthens the bond between client and caseworker.
6. Programs must be gender and culturally sensitive to retain women from a variety of racial and ethnic backgrounds. ■

Chapter 4

Conclusion

Addressing barriers to recruitment and retention of pregnant and parenting substance-using women into health and drug treatment programs requires creative and flexible approaches that can be modified if not effective. The 10 members of the PPWI focus group acknowledged the difficulties inherent in overcoming barriers, and emphasized that there is a lack of agreed-upon definitions of when in the process the client is considered to be either recruited or retained. The group came to consensus after considerable discussion, and developed agreed-upon definitions.

Before successful recruitment can take place, program staff must have a thorough understanding of the needs and lifestyles of substance-using pregnant and parenting women. Creating referral networks with other agencies was considered essential to recruiting substance-using pregnant and parenting women. Staff training on appropriate screening methods was critical to increasing the number of referrals. Various outreach methods were implemented to identify substance-using women in the community. This involved program staff going to locations where prospective clients were likely to spend time, including Laundromats, clinics, local WIC offices, beauty shops, and stores. A few programs sent outreach workers door to door. While some programs reported modest success with community outreach approaches, these activities were seen primarily as labor intensive and may not be cost-effective. Still, for hard-to-reach women using substances, there are few other approaches to reach them.

Cultural sensitivity to the ethnic backgrounds of the clients was critical to establishing substance abuse programs as a place where women would want to come. This included hiring staff who represented the ethnic backgrounds of the clients and who spoke their language. Programs must establish a sense of trust and understanding with clients before they can engage them in services.

Women who are addicted to substances live in a social environment where there is little long-term planning. This may include an inability to wait to access services, including treatment. Therefore, substance abuse programs must reduce the waiting time from initial contact to entry into program. Most of the programs in the focus group admitted clients immediately or within a few days. When programs were full, staff attempted to maintain contact with prospective clients.

Addressing child care and transportation needs was essential to successful recruitment. Providing incentives such as gifts to prospective clients was widely used by projects; however, the use of incentives did not appear to be a successful recruitment strategy. It may, however, have aided some programs in client retention.

Finally, it is essential that programs serving substance-using pregnant and parenting women conduct staff training to address attitudes about serving this population. The programs most successful at recruiting pregnant and parenting substance-using women provided extensive staff training, tried a variety of approaches, were flexible in altering approaches, and accepted clients on their own terms (e.g., delaying extensive intake forms until the client was emotionally ready).

The ability to retain women in substance abuse programs requires attention to several areas. First, the physical environment must appear homelike and safe to prospective clients. An emotionally safe and supportive environment allows women in treatment to address issues of sexual, physical, and emotional abuse at a rate appropriate for them. The therapeutic relationships that develop between clients and staff seemed to bond women to programs. Celebrating milestones and anniversaries empowered clients to remain drug free. Programs found it critical to address the long-term housing needs of women in treatment programs to retain them in programs. The members of the focus group agreed that providing incentives fostered client participation and improved retention rates.

While the environments where services to pregnant and parenting substance-using women are provided are changing rapidly due to managed care, it is still essential to ensure that high-risk pregnant and parenting women who use substances are being identified and provided drug treatment and other services to ensure healthy outcomes. Successful interventions resulting in recruitment and retention of substance-using pregnant and parenting women can lead to long-term cost savings as well as improved health for these women and their children. ■

References

1. National Institute on Drug Abuse. 1994. *National Pregnancy and Health Survey.* Rockville, MD: National Institute on Drug Abuse.

2. Chasnoff I. 1988. Drug use in pregnancy: Parameter of risk. *Pediatric Clinics of North America* 35:1403–1412.

3. Laken MP, Hutchins E. 1995. *Building and Sustaining Systems of Care for Substance-Using Pregnant Women and Their Infants: Lessons Learned.* Arlington, VA: National Center for Education in Maternal and Child Health.

4. Ewing H, Foran M. 1993. The role of prenatal care services in assisting families affected by drugs, alcohol, and AIDS. In R Barch, G Pietrzak, M Ramler, eds. *Families Living with Drugs and HIV: Intervention and Treatment Strategies.* New York: Guildford Press.

5. Boyd CJ. 1993. The antecedents of women's crack cocaine abuse: Family substance abuse, sexual abuse, depression and illicit drug use. *Journal of Substance Abuse Treatment* 10:433–438.

6. Hutchins E. 1995. *Psychosocial Risk Factors Associated with Drug Use During Pregnancy.* Unpublished doctoral dissertation. Johns Hopkins University, Baltimore.

7. Smith IE, Dent DZ, Coles CD, Falek A. 1992. A comparison study of treated and untreated pregnant and postpartum cocaine-abusing women. *Journal of Substance Abuse Treatment* 9:343–348.

8. Gehshan S. 1993. *A Step Toward Recovery: Improving Access to Substance Abuse Treatment for Pregnant and Parenting Women.* Southern Regional Project on Infant Mortality.

9. Goldsmith S. 1990. Prosecution to enhance treatment. *Children Today* July/August:13–36.

10. Adams C, Eyler FD, Behnke M. 1990. Nursing intervention with mothers who are substance abusers. *Journal of Perinatal and Neonatal Nursing* 3:43–52.

11. Poland ML, Ager J. 1990, April 23. Testimony for Hearings Before the Select Committee on Children, Youth, and Families. Detroit, MI: U.S. House of Representatives.

12. Chavkin W. 1990. Drug addiction and pregnancy: Policy crossroads. Public Health and the Law. *American Journal of Public Health* 80:483–487.

13. Breitbart V, Chavkin W, Wise P. 1994. The accessibility of drug treatment for pregnant women: A survey of programs in five cities. *American Journal of Public Health* 84:1658–1661.

14. Narrow WE, Regier DA, Rae DS, Manderscheid RW, et al. 1993. Use of services by persons with mental and addictive disorders. *Archives of General Psychiatry* 50:95–107.

15. Capaldi D, Patterson GR. 1987. An approach to the problem of recruitment and retention rates for longitudinal research. *Behavioral Assessment* 9:169–177.

16. Howard J. 1992. Subject recruitment and retention issues in longitudinal research involving substance-abusing families: A clinical services context. In *Methodological Issues in Epidemiological, Prevention, and Treatment Research on Drug-Exposed Women and Their Children* (NIDA Monograph 117). Rockville, MD: National Institute on Drug Abuse.

17. McCorkle R, Packard N, Landenburger K. 1984. Subject accrual and attrition: Problems and solutions. *Journal of Psychosocial Oncology* 2:137–146.

18. Young CL, Dombrowski M. 1989. Psychosocial influences on research subject recruitment, enrollment and retention. *Social Work Health Care* 14:43–57.

19. Moodley-Kunnie T. 1988. Attitudes and perceptions of health professionals toward substance use disorders and substance-dependent individuals. *International Journal of Addictions* 23:469–475.

20. Corse SJ, McHugh MK, Gordon SM. 1994. Enhancing provider effectiveness in treating pregnant women with addictions. *Journal of Substance Abuse Treatment* 12:3–12.

21. Schwarz RH. 1993. Not in my practice. *Obstetrics and Gynecology* 82:603–604.

22. Matera C, Warren WB, Moomjy M, Fink DJ, et al. 1990. Prevalence of use of cocaine and other substances in an obstetric population. *American Journal of Obstetrics and Gynecology* 163:797–801.

23. Zuckerman B, Frank D, Hingson R, et al. 1989. Effects of marijuana and cocaine use on fetal development. *New England Journal of Medicine* 320:762–768.

24. Sokol R, Ager J, Martier S. 1992. Methodological issues in obtaining and managing substance abuse information from prenatal patients. In *Methodological Issues in Epidemiological, Prevention, and Treatment Research on Drug-Exposed Women and Their Children* (NIDA Monograph 117). Rockville, MD: National Institute on Drug Abuse.

25. Khavari K, Douglass F. 1981. The drug use profile: An instrument for clinical research evaluations for drug use patterns. *Drug and Alcohol Dependency* 8:119–130.

26. Halpern R. 1992. Challenges in evaluating community-based health and social intervention: The case of prenatal care outreach. *Journal of Social Service Research* 16:117–131.

27. Poland ML. 1993. Practical approaches to outreach, maintenance, and followup. In *Pregnancy and Exposure to Alcohol and Other Drug Use.* CSAP Technical Report 7:61–68. Rockville, MD: U.S. Department of Health and Human Services.

28. Winick C. 1985. Specific targeting of prevention programs in alcohol and drug dependence. *International Journal of Addictions* 20:527–535.

29. Warrick LH, Wood AH, Meister JS, de Zapien JG. 1992. Evaluation of a peer health worker prenatal outreach and education program for Hispanic farmworker families. *Journal of Community Health* 17:13–26.

30. Bray ML, Edwards LH. 1994. A primary health care approach using Hispanic outreach workers as nurse extenders. *Public Health Nursing* 11:7–11.

31. Finlinson HA, Robles RR, Colon HM, Page JB. 1993. Recruiting and retaining out-of-treatment injecting drug users in the Puerto Rico AIDS prevention project. *Human Organization* 52:169–175.

32. Brown S, ed. 1988. *Prenatal Care: Reaching Mothers, Reaching Infants.* Washington, DC: National Academy Press.

33. Moras K. 1993. Substance abuse research: Outcome measurement conundrums. *NIDA Research Monograph* 137. Rockville, MD: National Institute on Drug Abuse.

34. Condelli WS. 1994. Predictors of retention in therapeutic communities. *NIDA Research Monograph* 144. Rockville, MD: National Institute on Drug Abuse.

35. Comfort M, Kaltenbach K, Smith A. 1995. Maternal psychosocial characteristics of pregnant cocaine dependent women: Residents vs. outpatients. Problems of drug dependence, 1994. In LS Harris, ed. *Proceedings of the 56th Annual Scientific Meeting, College on Problems of Drug Dependence. Vol. II, NIDA Monograph 153.* Rockville, MD: National Institute on Drug Abuse.

36. Lundy A, Gottheil E, Serota RD, Weinstein SP, et al. 1995. Gender differences and similarities in African-American crack cocaine abusers. In LS Harris, ed. *Proceedings of the 56th Annual Scientific Meeting, College on Problems of Drug Dependence. Vol. II, NIDA Monograph 153.* Rockville, MD: National Institute on Drug Abuse.

37. Shoptow S, Rawson R, Grella C, Anglin D, et al. 1995. Effectiveness of integrating enhancements to standard methadone treatment for subjects at high risk for HIV transmission. In LS Harris, ed. *Proceedings of the 56th Annual Scientific Meeting, College on Problems of Drug Dependence. Vol. II, NIDA Monograph 153.* Rockville, MD: National Institute on Drug Abuse.

38. Gainey RR, Wells EA, Hawkins JD, Catalano RF. 1993. Predicting treatment retention among cocaine users. *International Journal of Addictions* 26:487–505.

39. Collins JJ, Allison M. 1983. Legal coercion and retention in drug abuse treatment. *Hospital and Community Psychiatry* 34:1145–1152.

40. Pompi KF. 1994. Adolescents in therapeutic communities: Retention and posttreatment outcome. *NIDA Research Monograph 144*. Rockville, MD: National Institute on Drug Abuse.

41. Stevens AJ, Arbiter N. 1995. A therapeutic community for substance-abusing pregnant women and women with children: Process and outcome. *Journal of Psychoactive Drugs* 27:49–56.

42. Simpson DD. 1979. The relation of time spent in drug abuse treatment to posttreatment outcome. *American Journal of Psychiatry* 136:1449–1456.

43. Bale RN, Van Stone WW, Kuldau JM, Engelsing TMJ, et al. 1980. Therapeutic communities vs. methadone maintenance. A prospective study of narcotic addiction treatment: Design and one-year followup results. *Archives of General Psychiatry* 37:179–193.

44. Rounsaville BJ, Kleber HD. 1985. Psychotherapy/counseling for opiate addicts: Strategies for use in different treatment settings. *International Journal of Addictions* 20:869–896.

45. Orsini K. 1991. *Quality Assurance Report.* Report prepared for Spectrum Addiction Services, Inc.

46. Strantz IH, Welch SP. 1995. Postpartum women in outpatient drug abuse treatment: Correlates of retention/completion. *Journal of Psychoactive Drugs* 27:357–373.

47. Zlupko LN, Kauffman E, Dore MM. 1995. Gender differences in drug addiction and treatment: Implications for social work intervention with substance-abusing women. *Social Work* 40:45–54.

48. Streissguth AP, Glunta CT. 1992. Subject recruitment and retention for longitudinal research: Practical considerations for a nonintervention model. *NIDA Research Monograph 117.* Rockville, MD: National Institute on Drug Abuse.

49. Hutchins E. 1989. Outreach and retention strategies. In OSAP Special Report #1: Pregnant and Postpartum Women and Their Infants. U.S. Department of Health and Human Services, Office for Substance Abuse Prevention.

50. Stevens SJ, Glider PJ. 1994. Therapeutic communities: Substance abuse treatment for women. *NIDA Research Monograph 144.* Rockville, MD: National Institute on Drug Abuse.

51 Wasnick C, Schaffer B, Bencivengo M. 1980, September. The sex histories of fifty female drug clients. Paper presented at the National Alcohol and Drug Coalition, Washington, DC.

52. Gilligan C. 1982. *In a Different Voice.* Cambridge, MA: Harvard University Press.

53. Moise R, Kovach J, Reed B, Bellows N. 1981. A comparison of black and white women entering drug abuse treatment programs. *International Journal of Addictions* 17:350–370.

54. Lewis BF, Ross R. 1994. Retention in therapeutic communities: Challenges for the nineties. *NIDA Research Monograph 144.* Rockville, MD: National Institute on Drug Abuse.

55. Laken M, Ager J. In press. Effects of case management on retention in prenatal substance abuse treatment. *American Journal of Drug and Alcohol Abuse.*

56. Carise D, Forman R, Randall M. 1995. Effect of drug of choice, family involvement, and employer involvement on treatment completion rates

of substance abusers. In LS Harris, ed. *Proceedings of the 56th Annual Scientific Meeting, College on Problems of Drug Dependence. Vol. II, NIDA Monograph 153.* Rockville, MD: National Institute on Drug Abuse.

57. Lee JH, Svikis D. 1995. Enhanced program retention of perinatal substance abusers following patient incentive program. In LS Harris, ed. *Proceedings of the 56th Annual Scientific Meeting, College on Problems of Drug Dependence. Vol. II, NIDA Monograph 153.* Rockville, MD: National Institute on Drug Abuse.

58. Laken MA, Ager J. 1995. Using incentives to increase participation in prenatal care. *Obstetrics and Gynecology* 85:326–329.

Appendix A

PPWI Focus Group

October 26–27, 1995

Participants

Margery Brooks, M.H.A.
Community Substance Abuse Services
Department of Public Health
Fourth Floor
1380 Howard Street
San Francisco, CA 94103

Sally Carter, M.S.W., A.C.S.W., L.C.S.W.
Maternity Division Director
Oklahoma State Department of Health
Maternal and Infant Health Service
Room 703
1000 Northeast 10th Street
Oklahoma City, OK 73117-1299

Susan Cox, R.N.C., C.A.R.N., B.S.N.
Center for the Treatment of Pregnancy and Addiction
St. Peter's Medical Center
246 Eaton Avenue
New Brunswick, NJ 08901

Peggy Glider, Ph.D.
Executive Director
Quail Enterprises
3965 West Orangewood Drive
Tucson, AZ 85741

JoAnne Lutz, R.N.
Project Director
New Start Project/Sacred Heart Medical Center
675 West Broadway
Eugene, OR 97402

Susan McQuiston, Ph.D.
Bay Bright Program
Baystate Medical Center
140 High Street
Springfield, MA 01199

Lisa Potti, M.S.W.
Director
S.O.S. Crisis Center
Washtenaw Family Support Network
101 S. Huron Street
Ypsilanti, MI 48197

Stephen Ridley, M.H.S.
Medical College of Pennsylvania
Hahnemann University
Mailstop 447
Broad and Vine Streets
Philadelphia, PA 19102

Paula Roberts, C.S.W.
Social Work Supervisor
Department of Social Work Services
Columbia Presbyterian Medical Center
622 West 168 Street
New York, NY 10032

Elizabeth Toledo
Women's Chemical Dependency Coordinator
Hispanic Health Council
175 Main Street
Hartford, CT 06106

Facilitators

Ellen Hutchins, Sc.D., M.S.W.
Health Care Administrator
Maternal and Child Health Bureau
Parklawn Building, Room 18A-38
5600 Fishers Lane
Rockville, MD 20857

Marilyn Poland Laken, Ph.D., R.N.
Professor, Obstetrics and Gynecology
Department of OB/GYN, 5 South
Wayne State University
4707 St. Antoine
Detroit, MI 48201

NCEMCH Staff

Gayle Vandenberg, M.A.
Senior Project Associate
National Center for Education in Maternal and Child Health
Suite 701
2000 15th Street North
Arlington, VA 22201-2617

Valerie Gwinner, M.P.P., M.A.
Project Director
National Center for Education in Maternal and Child Health
Suite 701
2000 15th Street North
Arlington, VA 22201-2617

Appendix B
Program Descriptions

BayBright Program
Springfield, Massachusetts
Susan McQuiston

The BayBright Program was a five-year demonstration project funded in July 1990 to provide comprehensive case management services to cocaine-using pregnant and parenting women and medical/developmental follow-up to their infants. The project involved a collaboration between Baystate Medical Center, a private, nonprofit tertiary care hospital in Springfield, Massachusetts, and The Brightside for Families and Children, a child welfare center in West Springfield, Massachusetts. The target population consisted of economically disadvantaged women from the greater Springfield area (Hampden County) who used cocaine during pregnancy and their cocaine-exposed infants. Specific aims were to:

— Identify 250 cocaine-using pregnant women during the first two grant years
— Enroll at least 100 women and infants in the program for the three-year follow-up period
— Provide comprehensive case management
— Improve prenatal care among participants
— Reduce participants' prenatal and postnatal substance use
— Improve medical and developmental outcomes in the infants of cocaine-using women enrolled in the project

Two hundred thirty-eight women were identified and 142 women and 143 infants were enrolled in the project. The intervention involved provision of comprehensive case management to program participants using a continuous counselor model. Serial assessments of the medical and developmental status of the infants of program enrollees, from birth to three years postpartum, served as a secondary intervention, although this activity was more directly tied to outcome evaluation.

The evaluation design included individual difference (correlational) analyses and comparison of naturally occurring comparison groups within the total population of identified cocaine-using pregnant women. Data were collected from medical record reviews, reviews of activity logs summarizing day-to-day client-case manager contact, completion of substance use histories and substance use updates at specified intervals, and serial assessments of pediatric and developmental status.

CHANCES Project
Philadelphia, Pennsylvania
Stephen Ridley

CHANCES is a demonstration project that sought to demonstrate that medical, educational, and psychosocial interventions provided to substance-using and/or abusing pregnant and postpartum women might result in better birth outcomes and the development of more effective and positive parenting practices. CHANCES served women residing in the metropolitan Philadelphia area.

Clients were provided with medical interventions such as prenatal care, other obstetrics and gynecological services, birth control, urine drug screens, and HIV testing. Clients were provided with educational interventions such as life skills education/training, nutrition, parenting current events, and parent-child activity education groups. Participants were offered at least one individual psychotherapy session and two group psychotherapy sessions per week. Clients were helped to access the social services needed to support themselves, their families, and their recoveries.

Recruitment was accomplished through word of mouth in professional circles, informally by clients within their social systems, and through inservice trainings within the hospital system of our parent institution, Medical College of Pennsylvania and Hahnemann University Hospital. Recruitment was also accomplished via the creation of an informal network of human service agencies and workers within agencies that provided services to pregnant and parenting women and their families. That network consisted of the Treatment Program, External Treatment Providers, Shelter and Housing Agencies, Child Welfare and Its Contracted Agencies, Family Court and Child Advocates Legal Unit, and Education and Employment Programs.

Amity/Las Madres
Tucson, Arizona
Peggy Glider

Amity/Las Madres was a five-year CSAP project that began in July 1990 in Tucson, Arizona. The center was initially designed to be a short-term program for substance abuse counseling, assessments, and referrals. It evolved to become a comprehensive learning and resource center for both mothers and children. Women frequently were referred to Las Madres through the legal system, specifically Child Protective Services or Pima County Adult Probation. They could also be self-referred, or enter the program through referrals by social service agencies or other substance abuse agencies.

The women's portion of the Las Madres Center provided services such as parenting and health classes, seminars, videos, groups, workshops, and retreats. A computer lab and GED teacher were provided on-site. Issues of childhood, family dynamics, relationships, abuse, and friendship were part of the curriculum. Community resources were accessed for additional services women might need such as continuing education, job placement, medical attention, vocational training, food, housing, or clothing. Two 15-passenger vans transported mothers and their children to and from the center and to appointments during the day. Las Madres staff frequently provided moral support and case management for women involved in health, legal, or correctional systems. In-home follow up services were provided monthly or based on individual need. In addition, the women of Las Madres had opportunities to access the network of support that Amity offered seven days a week to individuals, families, and children, which included family groups and residential treatment.

The Children's Center was located in the same building as the women's center and was a fully licensed child care facility. There were three separate classrooms—infants, toddlers, and preschoolers—with children ranging in ages from birth to five years. The teachers were trained throughout the course of the grant to deal with special problems, such as developmental delays or behavioral difficulties. The length of the program was determined to be approximately one year, but varied considerably by individual need and commitment. Goals for participants included abstinence from drugs, development of parenting skills, ability to recognize and understand destructive patterns in relationships, building of friendships and support systems, completion of GED and/or enrollment in continuing education, resolution of legal matters, job training, life skills, and employment.

ADAPPT
Oklahoma City, Oklahoma
Sally Carter

The ADAPPT Project was a multilevel prevention and service coordination program that sought to improve and expand services throughout Oklahoma. ADAPPT served 1,897 substance-using women or women at risk for substance abuse of childbearing age primarily in areas of Lawton, Oklahoma City, Tahlequah, and Tulsa. ADAPPT focused on three goals:

1. Promote the involvement and coordinated participation of multiple organizations in the delivery of comprehensive services for substance-using pregnant women and their infants;
2. Increase availability and accessibility of prevention, early intervention, and treatment services for low-income women of childbearing age; and
3. Improve the birth outcomes of women who used alcohol and other drugs during pregnancy and decrease the incidence of infants affected by maternal substance use.

To achieve these goals, ADAPPT used these interventions:

1. Task forces were convened in three of the targeted communities;
2. Technical assistance was provided statewide free of charge;
3. Client identification techniques were developed and improved;
4. Case management was provided at all sites;
5. Professional and public education was conducted statewide; and
6. Evaluation of program activities was integrated with services.

The following results were achieved:

1. Referrals between agencies increased as a result of a coordinated and enlarged service delivery system;
2. Barriers to services were reduced through community action and case management funds;
3. Chemical dependency screening instruments identified target population better than interview;
4. Health care providers increased knowledge that would promote improved identification and quality of care;
5. Public awareness campaign increased requests for prenatal care;
6. Health risks including alcohol, tobacco, and other drug use were reduced through preconception counseling; and
7. Women receiving case management services received adequate prenatal care.

WINS
New York, New York
Paula Roberts

Women in Need of Services (WINS) is a comprehensive drug and prevention treatment program located in the Washington Heights/Inwood section of New York City. WINS serves a target population of low-income pregnant and postpartum women who use crack/cocaine. The program provides comprehensive services including: acupuncture treatment, individual and family counseling, group therapy, and HIV education/testing and case management, all of which are integral parts of the program. The program goal is to enable drug-addicted women with multiple psychosocial needs to care for their babies in the community, to prevent unnecessary foster care placement, and to become drug-free.

The WINS program provides comprehensive medical care, drug treatment, and social services on-site at Columbia-Presbyterian Medical Center. Being a part of a major medical center, the WINS program provides a "one-stop shopping" model of care. The Women, Children Care Center (WCCC) was specifically designed to meet the health and social service needs of HIV-infected and/or substance-abusing women and their children and family members. The WCCC offers primary obstetric, gynecologic, and pediatric care, along with specialized infectious disease medical care for seropositive newborns. Although the primary focus is substance abuse treatment, WINS also provides a one-stop shopping model integrating prenatal, postpartum, and pediatric care, psychiatric care, parent training, Narcotics Anonymous, nutritional guidance, and other related services.

SOS
San Francisco, California
Margery Brooks

The Support, Outreach, and Services (SOS) project is a collaborative effort of Community Substance Abuse Services and community-based organizations in response to the need to develop a comprehensive program for substance-using pregnant and postpartum women and their infants. SOS aims to provide early intervention, treatment, and support services to low-income women of color addicted to crack/cocaine residing in the Mission District and Bayview Hunter's Point areas of San Francisco. SOS is a drug-free outpatient model using a team approach to ensure coordination of outreach, case management, substance abuse treatment, and prenatal services to promote the shared goal of recovery and an optimal outcome for mothers, infants, families, and communities. The client and case manager develop an individual service plan. The case manager assists clients in recognizing their problems, and coordinates and monitors access to prenatal care, treatment services, health education and nutritional counseling, parenting and life skills training, child care, and transportation assistance. The drug counselor assists clients by providing education, support, and motivation for women making the transition from addiction to abstinence. She helps clients develop skills to reduce their dependence and establish a recovery lifestyle plan with emphasis on personal growth and family functioning. The case manager and drug counselor participate in case conferences to ensure overall service delivery and continuity of care. An important element of the project is the coordinated effort between staff and Department of Social Services/Child Protective Services (DSS/CPS) to maintain intact families and promote family reunification. In addition, the project provides outreach and education to individuals and communities on the issues of perinatal substance abuse and the availability of treatment alternatives and support services for substance-using pregnant and postpartum women.

CTPA
New Brunswick, New Jersey
Susan Cox

The Center for the Treatment of Pregnancy and Addiction (CTPA) is an outpatient substance abuse treatment program for pregnant and postpartum women and their children. Women may enroll in the program throughout their pregnancies and up to 90 days postpartum. Once enrolled, women may participate up to 18 months postpartum. CTPA provides services to central New Jersey (Middlesex and Somerset Counties).

Services provided include:

Substance Abuse Treatment: Individual counseling and five addiction groups, including psychoeducational and process groups, are provided each week. Drug-free and methadone-maintenance clients receive services together. Methadone is distributed through neighboring methadone-maintenance clinics. CTPA uses a 12-step philosophy.

Prenatal Care: Services are provided at St. Peter's Medical Center. Clients are followed by a CTPA coordinator providing direct patient care and maternal-fetal physicians.

Parenting Education: Clients attend one of three groups weekly. Individual counseling is provided as needed.

Nutrition: Weekly clients receive education while preparing a meal at "Lunch and Learn" sessions.

Social Work/Discharge Planning: Clients attend one of two groups weekly. Group topics include housing issues, child welfare, domestic violence, values clarification, welfare, Medicaid, WIC, food stamps, infant supplies, and clothing. Clients meet weekly with a clinical social worker.

Pediatrics: Enrollment of newborns and siblings in pediatric care. Home visits by an R.N. with NCAST assessments.

Child Care: Babysitting by child care attendant while mothers are on-site receiving services. Supervision by R.N.

Childbirth Education: A series of three classes is offered each month.

Outreach: Home visits by an outreach worker and community counselor.

MISAN
Detroit, Michigan
Lisa Potti

The Detroit Health Department's Mothers and Infants Substance Addiction Network (MISAN) is a demonstration project funded by the former Office of Substance Abuse Prevention for the three-year period September 1989 to August 1992. The purpose of the demonstration is to develop a continuum of care model to coordinate maternal and infant care with substance abuse treatment and to document its effectiveness.

MISAN coordinates substance abuse treatment and maternal and infant care for low-income substance-abusing pregnant women through a case management system designed to ensure that substance-abusing pregnant women receive the substance abuse treatment, prenatal care, and support services they need for healthy pregnancies.

To ensure early identification of substance-abusing pregnant women, a referral network was established with Hutzel Hospital's Eleonore Hutzel

Recovery Center (EHRC), the Detroit Health Department's Central Diagnosis and Referral Service (CDRS), and the 961-BABY hotline in Detroit.

The care management services offered by the MISAN program include: identification of barriers to attaining health services; assessment of needs in attaining and managing resources of daily living; assistance in appropriate use of health and human service agencies; assistance in establishing and maintaining client systems of social support; and assistance in identification and pursuit of client goals for education and employment,.

Each client receives an individual psychosocial and nursing assessment in her home. Following this, the case manager develops a treatment plan based on the client's expressed needs. Referrals to health and human service organizations are provided throughout the client's pregnancy and the first year of the infant's life. Follow-up visits and evaluations each month enable the case manager to alter the client's treatment plan as her needs change.

Follow-up support is provided to the mother after delivery to ease recovery from childbirth, to help her gain or maintain abstinence from drugs, and to facilitate her re-entry into a normal lifestyle. The infant is evaluated monthly by a public health nurse who monitors the child's growth and health to ensure that the child is receiving routine pediatric health care as well as care for specific health problems.

MISAN contracted with the Healthy Baby Van Service at the Detroit Health Department to provide MISAN clients with transportation for both prenatal care and substance abuse treatment. Case conference meetings between the MISAN staff and the staff at Eleonore Hutzel Recovery Center are scheduled once a month. These meetings enable the MISAN staff to ensure that the clients are participating in treatment, and to address client needs that have surfaced during treatment.

New Start
Eugene, Oregon
JoAnne Lutz

The primary goal of the New Start program is to identify and offer assistance to low-income women who are considered at risk for using alcohol and other drugs early in their pregnancies and to sustain their involvement with appropriate social, health, and substance abuse services. The community-based program relies on the coordinated efforts of local drug and alcohol treatment providers, as well as social and health service organizations, and is designed to decrease the incidence of infants affected by maternal substance use.

New Start staff encourage screening by private physicians and other prenatal care providers using the prenatal questionnaire developed by New Start to identify possible program members. Referrals from community social service agencies and treatment centers can be made directly by calling the New Start office. Self-referrals are also accepted.

Pregnant and/or postpartum low-income women at risk for substance abuse are in need of intensive outreach services. As a preventive program, New Start is designed to help women by providing them with a comprehensive support program that assists them in becoming drug-free during and after their pregnancies. New Start encourages its members in living a drug-free lifestyle by helping them acquire basic life skills pertaining to their pregnancies, mental health, and families. New Start provides an array of generic helping services through resource information and referral, mental health counseling, medical assistance, parenting education, and ongoing support for up to one year after the baby is born. New Start members are provided with an Intake upon entering the program and are continually assessed and counseled on issues involving their substance use and/or abuse. Chemical dependency treatment referrals are provided to New Start members and continual support and follow-up to these referral agencies are maintained and monitored. Pregnant women in the New Start program are considered at risk not only for substance abuse but also for a variety of other problems. New Start provides resource information and referral for medical, nutritional, financial, and counseling needs as well as housing, transportation, and child care support. Every member is provided with incentive vouchers to encourage ongoing New Start participation.

Cuidate Mujer
Hartford, Connecticut
Elizabeth Toledo

The Cuidate Mujer Program is a culture- and gender-specific prevention and treatment program for pregnant, postpartum, and childbearing-age Latina women in the Hartford area that consists of the following components:

- Prevention support group for women at risk for substance use; sessions are held on a weekly basis.

- Outpatient day treatment program based at Hartford Hospital that meets four days a week. Point of entry is through the case management component at the Hispanic Health Council.
- Mujeres Anonymous (12-step model) support group adapted to the Latina woman's needs; sessions are held on a weekly basis.
- Nuevos Pasos support group for women who have been in recovery for a specified period of time.
- Intensive case management that includes
  - Referrals to services such as treatment, housing, prenatal, postnatal, and medical, and legal
  - Home visits
  - Advocacy
  - Support
- Parent aide who offers assistance, education, and support on evenings and weekends to participants as a way to prevent child abuse/neglect among drug-exposed children and to prevent relapse among substance-using mothers.
- Pro Kids, offering regular prenatal screening, developmental assessment, and parent education for drug-involved women throughout their pregnancies and up to one year postpartum.
- Partners counselor who offers clinical therapy, education, and support for partners.
- Support services, transportation, child care, and snacks.
- Educational, cultural, and recreational activities.